| DATE DUE | |
|---|---|
| | |
| | |
| | |
| | |
| | |
| | |
| | |
| | |
| | |
| | |
| | |
| | |
| | |
| | |
| | |

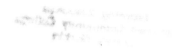

# HOME
# HEALTH CARE
# ADMINISTRATION

**Delmar Publishers' Online Services**

To access Delmar on the World Wide Web, point your browser to:

**http://www.delmar.com/delmar.html**

To access through Gopher: gopher://gopher.delmar.com

(Delmar Online is part of "thomson.com", an Internet site with information on more than 30 publishers of the International Thomson Publishing organization.)

For information on our products and services:

email: info@delmar.com

or call 800-347-7707

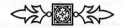

# HOME HEALTH CARE ADMINISTRATION

Susan Craig Schulmerich, RN, MS, MBA, CNA, CEN
Executive Director
Montefiore Medical Center Home Health Agency

Timothy J. Riordan, Jr., MBA
Chief Financial Officer
Montefiore Medical Center Home Health Agency

Stephanie Taylor Davis, RN, MS
Associate Executive Director
Montefiore Medical Center Home Health Agency

**Delmar Publishers**™
I(T)P **An International Thomson Publishing Company**

Albany • Bonn • Boston • Cincinnati • Detroit • London • Madrid • Melbourne
Mexico City • New York • Pacific Grove • Paris • San Francisco • Singapore • Tokyo
Toronto • Washington

# NOTICE TO THE READER

Cover Design: Carol D. Keohane

**Delmar Staff**
Publisher: Diane Mc Oscar
Acquisitions Editor: William Burgower
Assistant Editor: Hilary Schrauf/Debra Flis
Production Editor: Marah Bellegarde
Art and Design Coordinator: Timothy J. Conners
Editorial Assistant: Diane Biondi

COPYRIGHT © 1996
By Delmar Publishers
a division of International Thomson Publishing Inc.

The ITP logo is a trademark under license.

Printed in the United States of America

For more information, contact:

Delmar Publishers
3 Columbia Circle, Box 15015
Albany, New York 12212-5015

International Thomson Publishing Europe
Berkshire House 168-173
High Holborn
London, WC1V 7AA
England

Thomas Nelson Australia
102 Dodds Street
South Melbourne, 3205
Victoria, Australia

Nelson Canada
1120 Birchmont Road
Scarborough, Ontario
Canada, M1K 5G4

International Thomson Editores
Campos Eliseos 385, Piso 7
Col Polanco
11560 Mexico D F Mexico

International Thomson Publishing GmbH
Konigswinterer Strasse 418
53227 Bonn
Germany

International Thomson Publishing Asia
221 Henderson Road
#05-10 Henderson Building
Singapore 0315

International Thomson Publishing—Japan
Hirakawacho Kyowa Building, 3F
2-2-1 Hirakawacho
Chiyoda-ku, Tokyo 102
Japan

1 2 3 4 5 6 7 8 9 10 XXX 01 00 99 98 97 96 95

**Library of Congress Cataloging-in-Publication Data**
Schulmerich, Susan Craig.
     Home health care administration / Susan Craig Schulmerich,
  Timothy J. Riordan, Jr., Stephanie Taylor Davis.
        p.      cm.
     Includes bibliographical references and index.
     ISBN 0-8273-6508-X
     1. Home care services--Administration. 2. Home care services--
  United States--Administration.   I. Riordan, Timothy J.
  II. Davis, Stephanie Taylor.   III. Title.
RA645.3.S38   1995
362.1'4'068--dc20                                            95-21975
                                                                CIP

This book is dedicated with thanks and love to our families: Fred Schulmerich; Michael, Samantha and Christopher Davis; Josephine, Michael, Stephanie and Nicole Riordan.

# TABLE OF CONTENTS

# PREFACE

Home health care, or community health care, or visiting nurses all mean the same thing: professional care at home. Home care has undergone many changes, but one thing has remained constant; patients do better at home rather than in hospital beds. Consider the fact that the physician and hospital staff have limited insight into how patients interact in their own environments, and how those environments often affect the patient's ability to comply with treatment plans. Home health care is the missing link. The field staff become the eyes and ears of the physician and other health care professionals. The job can sometimes be physically hazardous and emotionally draining, but it is intellectually stimulating, and the unexpected can almost always be guaranteed.

This text is written for students, administrators, or professional staff new to home health care. As well, seasoned home health care administrators may find the text useful in shedding new insight on old problems. It is not designed to give "cookbook" answers to individual and unique issues, but rather to provide a foundation on which to build and develop planning strategies for the future management of home health care organizations. Home health care is the acknowledged wave of the future in the delivery of health services. It is dynamic, challenging, and one of the most interesting facets of health care.

The notion for this text was the result of one author's lack of experience in the delivery of home health services. The need to find a generic, comprehensive, easy to read reference on the subject of home health care administration was acute. However, no references were to be found. *Home Care Administration* is written to provide a general, but global, view of:

- General management
- Financial management
- Delivery of patient services
- Future trends

The *general management* section will discuss the history of home health care and universal information for any agency. Specific chapters will address: fundamental organization of an agency, regulatory considerations, empowering the work force, legal and risk management issues and, automation of an agency.

In *financial management* the basic tenets of the financial management of an agency will be explored and, the nuances of home care reimbursement will be addressed in detail.

*Delivery of patient services* will include discussions on recruitment of staff, organization for the delivery of services, relationships with referral sources, program development and, formation of professional standards.

*Future trends* may well become the actual environment by the time this text is published. In the United States, the delivery of health care, and the financing of that care are moving at a pace that leaves consumers, providers, and payers bewildered. In 1993, President Clinton's administration identified health care costs as the number two domestic issue to be tackled and brought under control; the economy was number one. These two issues are intimately intertwined, and yet, diametric to one another. Any student of health care economics will readily acknowledge that health care does not respond to normal market factors such as supply and demand and elasticity. How politicians and insurers propose to remedy the economic imbalance that plagues the industry is yet to be seen. Future Trends will discuss the "health care reform *d'jour*" and how it might effect the home care industry. *Case Studies* are highlighted throughout the book to reinforce the discussion.

The editor and authors wish to extend their appreciation to Ruth Alward who encouraged us to accept the challenge of writing this book. To the staff at Delmar, in particular Bill Burgower, Debra Flis, Hilary Schrauf, and Marah Bellegarde, for their patience and guidance in making this a reality. A special thanks to Fred Rosenstein, Vice President Corporate Programs, at Montefiore Medical Center (Bronx, NY) for his support and leadership. Our appreciation is extended to the reviewers for their constructive criticism and helpful suggestions. They include:

Thelma Domenici
Hospital Home Health
Albuquerque, NM

Carolyn Handler
National Hospital Alliance
Elmhurst, IL

Last, but far from least, to the contributing authors for their expertise and willingness to share it.

Susan Craig Schulmerich, Editor
Stephanie Taylor Davis
Timothy Riordan

# EDITOR'S BIOGRAPHY

Susan Craig Schulmerich, R.N., M.S., M.B.A., C.N.A., C.E.N. has been a practicing Registered Nurse since 1966. Prior to working at the Montefiore Medical Center Home Health Agency, Bronx, New York as the Executive Director, she held positions of staff nurse to Director of Operations in a number of hospitals in New York and Connecticut. Her experience included critical care, operating room, education, and emergency service.

After receiving a Diploma in Nursing from the Mount Vernon Hospital School of Nursing she successfully completed undergraduate requirements for a Bachelor of Science, Psychology at St. Thomas Aquinas College. A Master of Science Degree in Community Health Administration and Master of Business Administration were awarded from Long Island University. She is currently pursuing a Doctorate in Business.

Mrs. Schulmerich has published numerous articles and has been a contributing author to several books, and serves as a consulting and section editor for two national professional publications, the Journal of Emergency Nursing and the Journal of Nursing Administration. She is active in local, state and national home care organizations and serves on a variety of committees such as: the Advisory Board for Home Care of the *Society of Ambulatory Care Professionals* (a constituent unit of the American Hospital Association), the Annual Meeting Committee of the *National Association for Home Care,* and the Home Care Advisory Committee of the *Healthcare Association of New York State.*

Susan is married and lives with her husband Fred in Rockland County, New York. She enjoys a variety of sports and is especially fond of equestrian competition and events.

## SECTION AUTHOR BIOGRAPHIES

*Stephanie Davis, R.N., M.S.* is currently the Chief Clinical Officer at the Montefiore Medical Center Home Health Agency in the Bronx, New York. She graduated from the Hunter–Bellevue School of Nursing in New York City with a Bachelor of Science in Nursing and later was awarded a Master of Science Degree from Long Island University.

After working in neurosurgery at the Moses Division of the Montefiore Medical Center she joined the Home Health Agency as a Coordinator, later became an Administrative Nursing Supervisor, then the Director of Quality Management and Utilization Review, and assumed her current position in 1992. The Chief Clinical Officer is responsible for the patient care operations for an agency that has an average daily census of 1150 and 155 professional staff.

Stephanie lives in the Bronx with her husband, Michael and two children, Samantha and Christopher. She is currently exploring education in the field of counseling and development.

*Timothy J. Riordan, Jr.* has over 14 years financial health care experience and currently is the Associate Executive Director of the Montefiore Medical Center Home Health

Agency. Previous positions were held at the Visiting Nurse Service of New York as Director of Reimbursement and at Empire Blue Cross/Blue Shield as Senior Auditor. Mr. Riordan holds a Masters in Business Administration from Manhattan College and a Bachelors in Public Accounting from Fordham University.

Tim lives with his wife, Josephine, son Michael, and daughters Stephanie and Nicole in the Bronx, New York. Although an avid baseball fan he enjoys all competitive team sports.

# CONTRIBUTING AUTHOR BIOGRAPHIES

*George Dugan* has been Vice President of Employee Relations for the Montefiore Medical Center since 1988. He was Corporate Director of Training for ITT Corporation, Vice President of Administration for Hospital Affiliates International, and Vice President of Employee Relations for Picker Corporation. He received a Bachelor of Science degree from Cornell University College of Industrial and Labor Relations.

George lives in Connecticut with his wife and family.

*Robert Gunther, M.D., J.D.* attended the C-Tec University School of Medicine, Santo Domingo, completed a residency in pathology, and was licensed in Rhode Island in 1986 to practice medicine. He received his law degree from California Western School of Law in San Diego and was admitted to the bar in Florida (1979), New York (1987), Supreme Court (1982), and Federal Courts of Southern and Eastern Districts of New York and South Florida. Dr. Gunther specializes in medical malpractice litigation.

Bob lives with his wife, Keelyn and daughter Michaela in Rye, New York.

*Edward Kahn* is President of Kahn Systems, Inc., an EDP systems and management consulting firm located in Carmel, New York. He is also Vice-President of Datarus, Inc. a developer and marketer of computer software to the health care industry located in the Bronx, New York. With over 25 years experience in automated information systems, he was Director of Management Information Systems for Mt. Sinai Medical Center New York City and St. Luke's Hospital, Newburgh, New York. Mr. Kahn majored in Computer Science at the University of Pittsburgh and New York University.

Ed lives with his wife Lyn in New York City and Carmel, New York. He is an accomplished SCUBA diver, enjoys travel and the fine arts.

*Isadore Rossman, Ph.D., M.D.* has been the Medical Director of the Montefiore Medical Center Home Health Agency since 1949. A graduate of the University of Chicago Medical School with a Doctorate in 1937 and medical degree in 1942 he has published widely in the fields of home care and chronic illness. He edited the standard text *Clinical Geriatrics,* now in its third edition. Among various books for the laity his most recent *Looking Forward, A Medical Guide to Successful Aging* was published in 1989 and received rave reviews. He was formerly Director of the Bureau of Chronic Disease Control, New York City Department of Health, on the Advisory Council to the National Institute on Aging, and a past president of the American Geriatric Society.

# INTRODUCTION

In 1985, diagnosis related groupings (DRGs) became the universal payment method for reimbursement of acute health care facilities. Diagnosis related groupings were an attempt to curtail the upward spiral of health care spending. This method of payment was based on an episode of care rather than on a per diem basis. The prevailing premise was that there were no economic incentives to discharge patients from hospital beds under the "old" reimbursement system. Therefore, the methodology for reimbursement had to change in order to force economy. Under DRGs a particular diagnosis would have an average length of stay (LOS) and associated revenue assigned. Irrespective of the patient LOS, the acute care facility would be paid only the dollars assigned to the DRG. For instance, if a particular DRG had a reimbursement of $9,000 for a LOS of 10 days, and the hospital was able to discharge the patient in 7 days, the hospital would be permitted to keep the "money saved." Conversely, if the patient LOS was greater than 10 days the hospital would not be reimbursed for the additional days. Sounds simple. However, the concept was flawed, hospitals *do not admit or discharge patients, physicians do.* The negative economic consequences for protracted LOS were placed on the wrong provider of service. Hospitals found themselves between the proverbial rock and hard place, with the payers on one side and the physicians on the other. Hospitals were held accountable for safe discharge planning and reducing LOS without being able to affect either independently.

In order to survive, hospitals had to identify physician acceptable alternatives to "routine" recuperation in acute hospital beds. One viable and already existing alternative was home care. By whatever provider, hospital based or free standing, home health agencies could provide the skilled services necessary for the continued, safe care of the acutely ill patient at home. The benefits were immediately obvious. The hospital could safely discharge "sicker and quicker." For the most part, patients wanted to be at home in familiar and comfortable surroundings. And the home health care industry had the potential to flourish with an abundant referral base. Could this be a win/win/win situation? For a period it was. However the payers, in particular Medicare and Medicaid, found that the expected benefit of DRGs was not being fully realized because money was still hemorrhaging out of the tax coffers and into the health care industry. The facts that patients were "doing better" at home, and the aging and indigent populations were growing, were not taken into account. Only one logical bureaucratic conclusion could be drawn, there must be some form of abuse of the system.

In health care reimbursement there is an acknowledged phenomena: as Medicare goes, so go all payers. In 1985, Medicare put a tourniquet on the financially hemorrhaging appendage, home care benefits, and all other payers followed suit. The furor that followed and the outcome of the battle is a text unto itself. Suffice to say that the beneficiaries and providers were bloodied but not bowed, and the restoration of the home care benefits were realized in the settlement of the *Stagger's suit.* Although the home care industry was vindicated in the *Stagger's,* the damage had already been done. Agencies across the nation suffered financially, some irreparably, during the period of 1985 to 1988. Cash flow trickled at best, onerous paper burdens were placed on agencies, conflicting regulations and the interpretation of those regulations abounded, and field staff were looking elsewhere for employment. In general it was the "great depression in home health care."

Those agencies that were able to survive the depression have experienced unparalleled growth in the last five years. The future of home care, in all likelihood, is assured. As the delivery of health care migrates toward "alternate" systems and sites, home care is a natural to supplant hospitalization for the treatment of some acute and chronic diseases and illness. The home health industry is still in a growth phase and has many opportunities for employment of *displaced* hospital personnel, especially the professional groups.

As little as two decades ago, it was unthinkable that a ventilator dependent patient would be anywhere other than an Intensive Care Unit; to think such a patient would be at home was heresy! The idea that a patient receiving intravenous vasoactive drugs outside the walls of a hospital was pure fantasy. As technology continues to improve the safety and appropriateness of "high tech" outside the traditional hospital setting, home care will be the logical environment to care for and maintain patients requiring these services. As the "baby boomers" reach maturity, they will exercise their independence and determination to maintain self direction and control to the last possible opportunity. They will demand the right to stay at home in surroundings in which they are comfortable and safe. These are but a few examples and reasons that home care will continue to grow irrespective of what health care reform brings. Home care is dynamic and energized; it is the future.

# TABLES AND FIGURES

## TABLES

## FIGURES

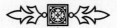

# PART ONE

## GENERAL MANAGEMENT

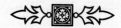

# CHAPTER

1

# Historical Overview of Community Health in the United States

Isadore Rossman
Susan Craig Schulmerich

# COMMUNITY ORIGINS

The history of community health care is a journey through the giving, caring, and nurturing nature of humankind. In small measure it also illustrates the frailty of egos and the danger of ignorance. Community health in the United States appears to have started in Charleston, South Carolina, in 1813. The Ladies Benevolent Society (LBS) was a group of wealthy gentlewomen who viewed the plight of blacks and poor whites as something that could not be tolerated in an enlightened society. To that end they adopted an organized program to feed, clothe, "nurse," and visit their charges (Buhler-Wilkerson, 1992). The LBS began its mission forty years before Florence Nightingale started her nursing career as superintendent for nursing at a home for gentlewomen on Harley Street (Widerquist, 1992). The Civil War would bring the abilities and talents of women to modern medicine. Caring for the wounded, maintaining hospital facilities in a condition acceptable for treating the wounded, and creating networks for the acquisition and procurement of necessary supplies were but a few of the impressive talents the women of the Ladies Aid Societies demonstrated. The United States Sanitary Commission, the precursor of the American Red Cross, was the official recognition by the government of the unique and necessary skills of women contributing to the health and safety of military personnel. At the close of the Civil War, the medical needs of the civilian population were numerous and the transition from wartime to peacetime aid was not that difficult (Tinkham, Voorhies, and McCarthy, 1984). Same enemy, different battlefield.

By 1886, the value of educated nurses and the contribution they could make to successful patient recovery was recognized. Middle and upper class patients benefited from this revelation. However, a new concept was gaining credit; the poor were entitled to the same care as the wealthy (Tinkham et al., 1984). It would seem the problem has not changed much in nearly 110 years!

In 1886, provision of care to the poor became the focus of two organized nursing districts, one in Philadelphia and one in Boston. The districts were separate and distinct from each other, but had common threads. First, they were started by women. Second, the women had been influenced by Englishman William Rathbone, who first introduced the theory of organized nursing districts (Tinkham et al., 1984). In 1893, Lillian Wald and Mary Brewster joined forces to create the Henry Street Nursing Settlement, which is now the Visiting Nurse Service of New York. Lillian Wald is credited for originating a three word description of the work the Henry Street Nursing Settlement did . . . *public health nursing* (Denker, 1993).

In the midst of the 1893 depression, the worst the nation had ever experienced, Wald and Brewster were continually confronted with disease, vermin, poverty, and filth in the tenements they visited. Realizing they could not fight, much less win, this battle alone, they enlisted the aid of private relief agencies and local medical entities to augment what the visiting nurses were doing. Wald's resourcefulness made it possible for sterilized milk, meals, and medicines to be provided free of charge to many of the sick and indigent. The role of the public health nurse began to expand well beyond caring for the sick—

prevention of illness and disease became a focal point. The Board of Health had vested in Wald and Brewster authority to improve the health of the neighborhoods they served. The women began crusades to clean rooftops and tenement hallways. It became obvious, however, that cleanliness was not the solution to the ever growing problem of illness and infection; Wald believed employment was a key ingredient in overcoming the devastation of illness she witnessed on a day-to-day basis. The role of the public health nurse was extending beyond simply visiting the sick, and expanding to embrace the physical, emotional, and economic health of the community (Denker, 1993).

After more than a decade and a half of experience in public health nursing, Wald theorized that insurance companies could reduce the disbursement of death benefits if patients who were home could receive skilled nursing care for illnesses and diseases that previously had been thought hopeless. Contracting with insurance companies "for a modest fee" was also a way in which the Henry Street Settlement could begin to support itself. Metropolitan Life Insurance Company (MetLife) agreed to test the assumption on June 1, 1909. Within three months the benefits were evident. So evident, in fact, that by 1916 approximately *9.4 million policyholders in 2,000 cities* had visiting nurse services available as part of their policies. Between 1909 and 1952, *one billion* home visits were made to MetLife beneficiaries (Denker, 1993).

Public health nursing, also known as *community health nursing*, remained in the charitable sector until 1947 when New York's Montefiore Hospital became a provider of community home care.

# HOSPITAL-BASED HOME CARE

Wars, economic depressions, industrialization, and a variety of other social factors influenced the growth of public health nursing. It took decades before hospitals would become involved in community care. One hospital with a rich and well known commitment to its social mission was, and still is, Montefiore Medical Center in the Bronx, New York. Hospital-based home care delivered by a multidisciplinary team was the vision of then hospital director Eli M. Bluestone, M.D. In contrast to the general opinion that the home was a rudimentary medical environment, old-fashioned, and retrogressive, Bluestone saw the home as a potential extension of the medical facility. A flexible view of the role, responsibilities, and capabilities of the modern hospital, accenting hospital-based home care, was pioneered by Bluestone.

Those who led Montefiore's home care were determined that there should be no decline in the quality of care, and that no one could ever assert that patients had been discharged from the hospital to an obviously inadequate alternative. Apart from contracted nursing services (initially, skilled nursing service was provided through the Visiting Nurse Service of New York) the home care program was set up to parallel the important basic services of the hospital: attending physicians, social workers, and physical and occupational therapists, all drawn from the staff of the hospital. Additionally, the chief of the neoplastic service and teaching cardiologists made periodic consultative rounds on the homebound patients. Initiated with grants from the New York Heart Association and the American Cancer Society, patients with cancer and cardiovascular disease were the first on the program (Rossman, Eger, and Cherkasky, 1950; Rossman, 1954). The Home Care Department, because it was part of the hospital, had access to beds, wheelchairs, and other durable medical equipment. The occupational therapist, doubling as an environmentalist, made a home visit prior to the patient's discharge to ascertain what the problems in the home environment might be and to review the equipment needs with the family.

It was not accidental that home care of this type originated at Montefiore (Bluestone, 1971). At that time it was titled Montefiore Home and Hospital for Chronic Disease. Some of the patients had been there for *years, even decades.* In addition to this base of long-term chronic illness, other patients with shorter-term illness required new technologies and specialized services; acute care beds were in demand. Not surprisingly, therefore, Montefiore had a well-deserved reputation for accepting patients with illnesses of indeterminate duration, including patients who were certainly terminal, or with disorders so disabling that reversibility was unlikely.

Naturally, a facility of this kind, with its accent on chronic disease, played an important part in the medical chain. There was a constant waiting list for admission. *Acute* hospitals were not eager to admit or readmit chronic patients. Hospitalization insurance often expired within twenty-one days, and generally was not available after age sixty-five. It was an unfortunate fact that many patients on the waiting lists died in the referring facility or at home.

These factors contributed some impetus to the development of the home care program at Montefiore. Those at Montefiore saw many chronic illnesses, and it was clear that there were phases not requiring continued hospitalization for adequate care (Cherkasky, 1949). Indeed, as was the custom then, some of these chronically ill patients had weekend passes to go home, further blurring the lines that defined the attributes of hospitalization. Thus the social service and nursing departments were highly aware of the needs of both short- and long-term care patients and their families. Given this set of circumstances it was inevitable that Montefiore would launch the hospital-based home care movement.

## PATIENT RESPONSES TO HOME CARE

Despite the heavy bias built into patient selection for home care, initially cancer and cardiovascular disease, some did show unexpected improvement at home. Forecasts of life expectancy emanating from hospital experts turned out to be erroneous. Prognoses of an undeviating downhill course were inaccurate. As the home care programs enlarged to encompass a greater variety of illnesses, it became clear that the home could be a therapeutic environment for some patients, in some ways superior to the hospital or institutional facility (Rossman, 1956).

A multifactorial, in-depth assessment of a home-treated and a control population would be required to prove this. As is clear retrospectively, such a study would have to call for psychiatric assessments of patients and families before and after home care. Necessary instrumentalities for such assessment would have to include: evaluation of depression and anxiety; study of patient and family expectations; study of diet and nutrition; evaluation of medications and their effects; and both the obvious and more subtle behavioral characteristics of the patient, family, and home care team. Such studies, which have never been done, would be formidable and costly.

What was done, and is by no means a minor measuring rod, was the clinical evaluation of the patient while in the hospital and after being on home care. Such clinical evaluations may be subject to bias in interpretations, but are not without merit. A ten pound weight gain, a decline in need for narcotics, or the abolition of episodes of pulmonary edema are indeed clinical facts. Clinical observations in the early years of home care indicated that some patients responded surprisingly positively to the new home environment.

# LASTING EFFECTS OF MONTEFIORE'S DEMONSTRATION

Home care turned out to be a major exploration into alternatives to institutional care, embracing far more than traditional public health nursing. Additionally, with the patients serving as their own caretakers, it somewhat unexpectedly illuminated the pros and cons of hospital care. It examined and reaffirmed the care giving potential of the family and home setting. From the viewpoint of delivery of care, it demonstrated that patients fell into a spectrum, with some complexities often defined by social and emotional rather than medical factors. Perhaps the most important part of the home care legacy was the sharpened focus on what defines the hospital patient. From this experience there flowed in later years such innovative concepts as hospice, after care programs, and, for better or worse (observers differ), *diagnosis-related groupings (DRGs)*.

Home care has demonstrated conclusively that patients, both acute and chronic, who would ordinarily continue in hospitals, could be as well served in home settings (Rossman, 1973). Some observers thought it possible that Montefiore was inhabited by patients who had somehow been uniquely preselected for home care. This was shown not to be the case a number of years after the genesis of hospital-based home care at Montefiore. Columbia Presbyterian Hospital in Manhattan permitted a home care physician and a social worker from Montefiore to conduct an evaluation of patients and families for appropriateness for admission to a home care program. The same criteria used for evaluating Montefiore patients were used again. The results indicated that 12 to 14 percent of patients on comparable services could have been sent home to a Montefiore-type home care program (unpublished data, Montefiore Hospital Home Health Agency, 1954).

With experience, it became clear home care was teaching a fundamental lesson to care givers and care planners that the concept of home care had wide and far-reaching applicability. For example, it could be used to reduce the length of stay for many acute medical or surgical illnesses. As the hospital day grew increasingly expensive, early discharge to home care became financially more attractive and finally imperative. Thus by the 1960s, some home care services had been added to many standard Blue Cross/Blue Shield contracts.

Economic factors continue to play an increasing role as the discussion of health care's high cost has escalated over recent years and is now on the forefront of the national political agenda. Power and control of one's fate has now shifted from the formerly autonomous hospital to the fiscal authorities. Thus the use of DRGs propelled hospitals into acceptance of home care—even if bed occupancy was low. And, as was discovered in the early years of the home care movement, the life and death of the movement is still controlled by the question of *fiscal anemia*.

With the passage of the decades, however, there has developed an unshakable conviction that home care, in some form, makes great financial sense. This is evidenced by the impressive growth in the number of home care agencies in the United States—7,400 (*Advance Data No. 256, 1994*). The country has entered into a cost cutting economy, but even at that, home care's durability is assured. As predicted many years ago, ". . . there is new emphasis on primary care and the training of primary care internists and family practioners. There is in the offing, legislation both at federal and state levels designed to encourage community care programs which will be supportive of the chronically ill and the elderly in a home environment. The success of home care such as ours, the unmet needs that have been fulfilled, and the institutional costs that have been saved make these programs and other alternatives harbingers of the future. If we are not driven in the home care direction by compassion, then we will be by fiscal pressure" (Rossman, 1977).

## CONCLUSION

The history of home care speaks well to the positive effects that *care at home* has on the well-being of the patient and the maintenance of the family unit's integrity. As the United States moves toward some type of health care reform, it would seem wise to evaluate the physical, emotional, and monetary benefits that home care brings to patients, families, payers, and society in general.

## REFERENCES

Bluestone, E.M. (1951, April). Some advantages of an extra-mural hospital program. *Hospital Management,* 71:18.

Buhler-Wilkerson, K. (1992). Caring in its proper place: race and benevolence in Charleston, S.C. 1813–1930. *Nursing Research,* 41(1):14–20.

Cherkasky, M. (1949). The Montefiore Hospital Home Care program. *American Journal of Public Health*, 39, 163.

Denker, E.P. (Ed.). (1993). *Healing at home: Visiting Nurse Service of New York 1893–1993*. New York: Visiting Nurse Service of New York.

Rossman, I., Eger, S.D., & Cherkasky, M. (1950). The treatment of cardiac patients on a home care program. *Modern Concepts of Cardiovascular Disease*, 19:7.

Rossman, I. (1954). Treatment of cancer on a home care program. *Journal of the American Medical Association*, 156:827.

Rossman, I. (1956). Reduction of anxiety in a home care setting. *Journal of Chronic Disease*,14:643.

Rossman, I. (1973). Alternatives to institutional care. *Bulletin of the New York Academy of Medicine*, 49:1084.

Rossman, I. (1977). Long term home care of chronic illness. *Clinical Medicine*. Unpublished data. Montefiore Medical Center Home Health Agency, 1954.

Tinkham, C.W., Voorhies, E.P., & McCarthy, N.C. (1984). *Community health nursing evolution and process in the family.* Norwalk, CN: Appleton-Century-Crofts.

U.S. Department of Health and Human Services. (1994). *Advance Data No. 256.* Hyattsville, Md.

Widerquist, J.G. (1992). The spirituality of Florence Nightingale. *Nursing Research*, 41(1) 49–55.

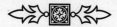

# CHAPTER

# General Information

**Susan Craig Schulmerich**

Home health care is a complex, convoluted, and sometimes thoroughly confusing aspect of health care delivery. It is one of the most intriguing and rewarding areas for clinical practioners, as well as a challenge for seasoned administrators who try to apply hospital process and practice in the arena of home care. There is a core of generic information that applies to home care no matter what state(s) the agency is licensed to practice in. This chapter will review the basics. The reader is encouraged to explore the peculiarities and nuances for the state in which they practice.

# AGENCY TYPES

Home care agencies can be freestanding, hospital-based, public, charitable, or a combination of any of the aforementioned. Freestanding agencies are independent and have no formal reporting lines to other organizations or entities. Hospital-based agencies are a department or division of a hospital, hospital consortium, or hospital network. Public agencies are generally affiliated with, sponsored by, and/or operated by a governmental agency such as the Public Health Department. Charitable organizations, usually religious in nature, are the fourth type of agency. Any of the agency types can exist in combination; for instance, the Health and Hospital Corporation (HHC) of the City of New York is a public organization that has hospital-based home care agencies in a number of the eleven acute care hospitals that comprise the HHC.

## Increase in Home Health Agencies

The growth of home care agencies has been striking. In 1965, there were 1,753 Medicare (M/C) certified agencies; in February of 1993, certified agencies numbered 6,497 (*Homecare News,* 1993). Hospital-based and proprietary agencies experienced the largest growth after the clarification of coverage settled by the *Staggers Suit* in 1987. The Staggers suit corrected the subjective, inconsistent interpretation of the Medicare benefit for home care service by the various regional intermediaries. Reported by the National Association for Home Care (NACH) in *Basic Statistics About Home Care 1993,* the number of home care agencies is represented in Table 2.1, Agency Inventory. *Certified* represents M/C certified home health agencies, *Hospice* are only those with M/C home care certification, and *Other* represents all noncertified hospice and home health agencies.

**TABLE 2.1** Agency Inventory

| *Certified* | *Hospice* | *Other* | *Total* |
|---|---|---|---|
| 6,497 | 1,223 | 6,231 | 13,951 |

In 1983, M/C added hospice to the benefit package. M/C certified hospices in January, 1984, numbered thirty-one; in nine years the providers of M/C certified hospice care have increased an average of 133 per year.

# PROGRAMS

An agency can be either for-profit or not-for-profit. It can be private (voluntary) or public. Regardless of the status, there must be a board of trustees responsible for the comprehensive management of the agency. And, as is usual practice today, the organization will be accredited by some independent certifying body, such as the Joint Commission for Accreditation of Healthcare Organizations (JCAHO) or the Community Healthcare Accreditation Program (CHAP).

## Certified Home Health Agency (Certified Agency)

The term certified is indicative of the receipt of *direct* reimbursement under Title XVIII and XIX (Medicare [M/C] and Medicaid [M/A] respectively) of the Social Security Act. The Health Care Financing Administration (HCFA) promulgates the rules and regulations, also known as the conditions of participation (COPs), for certified agencies. Each state may also generate its own rules and regulations, but they cannot be less stringent than the federal COPs if the agency is to be recognized as certified. The state may *choose* to duplicate the federal COPs as its basis for licensing requirements.

### Qualifications for Admission to a Certified Program

The length of stay (LOS) in a certified program is expected to be short; the COPs dictate whether the patient requires *intermittent, skilled, finite,* or *restorative care.* Intermittent means that prolonged "round-the-clock" nursing or aide care cannot be provided. Skilled indicates that the patient has a need for professional care from one of three *qualifying* services of nursing, physical therapy, or speech therapy. Finite is interpreted to mean that there is an expected end to the care (death is not acceptable) and that restorative, not maintenance or custodial, care is required. This by no means is an exhaustive description of a certified agency but can be used for comparison to the definitions of other types of agencies.

## Long-Term Home Health Care Programs (LTHHCP)

In 1975, New York experienced a severe shortage of skilled nursing facility (SNF) beds, known at that time as nursing home beds, that caused no end of difficulties for the acute care hospitals. Bottlenecks in emergency departments and the canceling of elective surgical procedures were just two of the operational problems facing the hospitals as they held patients who were candidates for SNF placement in acute hospital beds. In 1978, in an attempt to partly relieve the shortage of SNF beds, the State of New York was granted a waiver to provide M/A reimbursement for otherwise nonreimbursable services under Title XIX. In a capsule, the program was designed to allow M/A recipients who did not meet admission requirements for a certified program to remain in their homes and receive services that previously were only available through an SNF. The LTHHCP in New York has become a model for other states and programs in delivering *traditional* institutional care.

The LTHHCP may become a matter of history by the time this text is published. In November of 1994, the voters in the state of New York sent a clear message to Albany (the state capital)—stop spending taxpayer dollars on rich entitlement programs. Newly elected Governor George Pataki (Republican) pledged to cut $5 billion in spending. One of the hardest hit will be the M/A program—$1.2 billion *in one year.* Slated to be dismantled, with ninety days notice, is the LTHHCP. Albeit fully understood that the LTHHCP is a cost efficient and humane program, the governor and his fiscal advisors believe that since other states care for the elderly in a less costly fashion, New York should emulate them. If in fact the LTHHCP becomes a matter of history, it will be a challenge to the health care delivery system in the state to care for the nearly 20,000 patients currently on the program.

### Costs and Services Available to LTHHCP Patients

In order to qualify, patient service consumption must be 75 percent or less than the cost of regional SNF placement; this is referred to as the *cap.* Exceptions to the caps are permitted, but by far the majority of LTHHCP patients are under the cap.

Aside from the services available to certified cases, LTHHCP provides an array of benefits such as transportation, meals, and housing improvement, just to name a few. Maintaining the frail elderly in the comfort, safety, and familiarity of their own homes is not only benevolent and dignified, but cost effective. If long-term home care becomes a reality under health care reform, New York State's successful experience could serve as a model for these new benefits.

## Noncertified Agencies

Noncertified agencies are not eligible for *direct* reimbursement under M/C or M/A. However, by contracting services to certified agencies, noncertified agencies receive significant dollars from M/C and M/A. These agencies can and do provide nursing, home health aide, personal care, or other services to patients through direct private pay or nongovernment payers. Licensure of noncertified agencies runs the gamut of nearly nonexistent rules and regulations for licensure to very stringent oversight by state authorities.

Some certified agencies *spin off* noncertified agencies or companies. The rationale for developing this business structure makes sense. If the certified agency must contract for paraprofessional or private duty service, why not purchase it from within your own system? It also makes sense from a *continuum of care* point of view. Patients who are no longer eligible for certified care, regardless of the reason, can be transferred to the non-certified company, if that is the appropriate venue for care. By transferring the patient within the *system,* the agency keeps the patient within the system. This becomes a positive selling point in negotiating with managed care organizations (MCOs) as well—one stop shopping. An additional benefit of a certified agency operating the noncertified company is that of quality control and management.

Although ineligible for direct government reimbursement, in 1991 HCFA promulgated home health aide competence requirements for the education and certification of home health aides (personal care workers) trained and employed by noncertified agencies. In effect this began federal regulation of this sector of home care.

## Home Medical Equipment

Home medical equipment (HME) is the generic identifier for respiratory therapy (RT) equipment and durable medical equipment (DME). Respiratory therapy equipment includes oxygen and associated apparatus, humidifiers, nebulizers, ventilators, tracheostomy supplies, and so on. Durable medical equipment is items such as beds, bathroom aides, walkers, and such. Hospital medical equipment is a primary support service to certified agencies, LTHHCPs, and noncertified programs in fulfilling the physician-ordered plan of care (POC). The advances in technology and the improvement in safety of technical equipment have led to making the home an extension of what was once only found in an intensive care unit. Reimbursement for the various components of HME is confusing at best. For the most part, M/C will pay for RT but will pay little to nothing for DME. Individual states vary in the *richness* of benefits for M/A recipients in the arena of RT or DME. Payers, other than the government, cover the spectrum of payment schedules. Usually HMEs bill directly to the payers.

Just as a certified agency can own and operate a noncertified agency, it can do the same with a HME. The benefits are the same in all respects.

## High Tech

The high technology (high tech) industry continues to experience impressive growth. High tech is usually defined as home infusion (including home intravenous [IV] antibiotic, chemotherapy, or blood component infusion), parenteral or enteral nutrition, high risk prenatal monitoring, and phototherapy. As more technologic and pharmacologic interventions become safer, such as IV administration of vasoactive drugs (pharmacologic agents that have an effect on the cardiovascular system, such as increasing the volume of blood the heart ejects with each beat), the incidence of home use will continue to grow.

Reimbursement for high tech service is even more poorly defined than HME. For the most part, it is paid for on a case-by-case basis. Reimbursement for service is usually negotiated when the case is initially reviewed and approved by the payer. Had federal health care reform (1993–1994) become a reality, the impact on availability of high tech services in the home would probably have been positive, but that appears to be a closed issue. However, the cost of health care continues to be a concern, and utilization of costly hospital beds is at the forefront of that concern. Methods and means to further reduce hospital LOS continue to gain favor. One such method is to provide home infusion for an ever expanding group of parenteral pharmacologic agents.

Again, a certified agency can create an infusion company to complete the complement of home health care services for patients and payers alike. In the era of vertical integration and associated economies, it makes a great deal of business sense to offer the spectrum of home health care needs through one organization.

# PAYERS

All payers have experienced an increase in expenditures for home care as a result of the prospective payment system (PPS) of diagnosis related groupings (DRGs). In 1985, PPS replaced traditional retrospective hospital reimbursement methodology. Prospective payment was expected to

1. stem the flow of dollars hemorrhaging from the insurance carrier and public coffers
2. limit the upward spiral of the cost of health care inflation
3. promote efficiency and effectiveness in what was thought to be an unreasonably costly delivery system

Prospective payment did in fact reduce hospital costs by reducing LOS, but it did not reduce the overall cost of health care—money was simply being spent in other venues. One of these was, and is, home care.

## Medicare

Medicare is by far the most comprehensive and best defined of all payers. Skilled, intermittent home care has been part of M/C benefits since its inception in 1965. However, as a result of the Omnibus Budget Reconciliation Act of 1980 (OBRA-80), the access to home care by M/C beneficiaries was enhanced by reducing or eliminating some of the more onerous reimbursement restrictions that had existed between 1965 and 1980. For instance

- relaxation of the number of days a beneficiary could receive home care services
- no prior hospitalization required
- particular therapy visits (physical and speech) permissible without skilled nursing as part of the plan of care (*National Medical Expenditures Home Health Care,* 1993)

In fact, between 1974 and 1986 there was a fourfold increase in the number of M/C patients receiving home care service and an average annual increase of twenty-four percent spent on home care benefits. In 1987, half of the six million people on home care were sixty-five years or older (*National Medical Expenditures Home Health Care,* 1993).

Medicare will reimburse a certified agency for

- skilled nursing
- physical, occupational, and speech therapy
- medical social work
- selected HME (provided either directly by the certified agency or through contract with a HME vendor)
- home health aide (provided either directly by the certified agency or through contract with a noncertified program)

## Medicaid

The Omnibus Budget Reconciliation Act of 1981 (OBRA-81) would bring to M/A home care benefits package what OBRA-80 brought to M/C. One exceptionally far-reaching result of OBRA-81 was the redirection of M/A long-term care from institutions to the community—the genesis of *long-term home health care* (see LTHHCP previously discussed). Between 1977 and 1986, M/A recipients benefiting from various pieces of legislation, such as OBRA-80, were 60 percent, compared with the fourfold increase in M/C. However, overall M/A spending increased sevenfold during the period (*National Medical Expenditures Home Health Care,* 1993).

Since M/A is administered through individual state design, the breadth and scope of coverage vary from state to state. As a general rule of thumb, with the exception of medical social work, the services covered and defined under M/C are paid for on the state level. In some states, the number of visits or hours of service may be limited or have a maximum utilization threshold (MUT). Or, in other instances, the M/A benefit for home care may be more liberal than M/C.

## Commercial Payers

Benefits for home care services cover the spectrum of zero to 100 percent of published charges, with no restrictions. Although the latter is unusual, it does exist. Commercial payers may set a limit on visits, dollars, time periods, or any combination thereof. There may be a burdensome prior approval process and an ongoing approval mechanism. The conflicts that arise when the certified agency believes the patient requires additional care and the payer is in disagreement is a professional and billing nightmare. The certified agency may find itself in a no-win situation. State regulations may forbid the discharge of a patient because of inadequate or no-payment stream, and the carrier simply can refuse to pay for any further service. In most cases there are grievance procedures, but they are typically time consuming, overly protracted, and adversarial.

## Managed Care

The term managed care is really a misnomer; it would be more accurate if it were called *managed finance of care.* How health care reform will affect managed care remains to be seen. However, health maintenance organizations (HMOs) and preferred provider organizations (PPOs) are in existence today, and all practice varying degrees of managed financial care for their participants. The focus of any HMO or PPO is to keep the subscriber (patient) well, which is an admirable goal. But should a subscriber become ill, then it is the goal of the organization to provide *safe* care in the most cost efficient manner. Subscribers are required to seek care from participating providers. The provider network covers the spectrum of health care services, from hospital to home care agency, pharmacy to physician, and HME to high tech. The financial consequences for not using the participating provider(s), when they exist in the network, can be impressive. However, there is no financial consequence for the patient *going outside* the provider network if the network cannot provide the necessary care.

Managed care arrangements for home care service generally require prior approval. The managed care organization will decide what will and will not be provided. If the home care agency believes a precarious medical legal situation exists because the managed care organization will not authorize adequate care and resources for the patient, it should seek legal counsel.

## Uncompensated Care

Depending on the state, bad debt and charity care may share the same definition or may be distinctly different, but the bottom line is, the care is *uncompensated.*

### Bad Debt

Bad debt is the failure of a patient, or payer, to pay for services rendered. The reason for failure to pay is of no consequence. Irrespective of the payer, an agency must make a good-faith effort, indicated by documented attempts, to collect the unpaid balance, before *writing off* the account. In some states there is a *bad debt pool* that assists health care organizations in offsetting some financial losses from unusual and/or extraordinary bad debt. For instance, in states where there is a disproportionately high number of undocumented aliens, the bad debt for health care can be devastating for providers. The bad debt pool would ameliorate some of the loss by making a year-end adjustment of revenue.

### Charity Care

On the other hand, charity care is provision of service to a patient who has no insurance, no means to pay for the service, and has a family income that is less than 200 percent of the federal poverty level. In New York a certified *agency must* annually provide 2 percent of its operational budget in charity care. Budgeting for charity care is a *moving target.* As census and associated costs of operating fluctuate, so does the amount to be devoted to charity care. It is wise to analyze the amount spent on charity care on at least a quarterly basis to make adjustments as necessary. A more in-depth treatment of payment sources can be found in Section II Finance beginning with Chapter 9.

# CONCLUSION

The *business* of home health care, as should have become evident while reading this chapter, shares some similarities with basic health care delivery systems. But the similarities are simply a starting point from which to build a knowledge base of the distinctions and differences that exist between home care and the rest of the industry. Much of what becomes the home care administrator's *common knowledge* is learned on the job. Unfortunately, some of the lessons can be costly and time consuming. It is recommended that the reader review the suggested readings to further expand awareness and understanding of the home care sector.

# REFERENCES

National Association for Home Care. (1993). *Basic statistics about home care 1993.* Washington, D.C.

National Association for Home Care. (1993). *Homecare news,* research update. Washington, D.C.

U.S. Department of Health and Human Services. (1993). *National medical expenditure survey home health care: use, expenditures, and sources of payment,* research findings 15. Washington, D.C.

## *Suggested Reading*

Buckley, T. (1993). Hospital-Based Home Medical Equipment Companies, *Hospital home care strategic management for integrated care delivery.* Chicago: American Hospital Association.

Lerman, D. & Linne, E. (Eds.). (1993). *Hospital home care strategic management for integrated care delivery.* Chicago: American Hospital Association.

United Hospital Fund of New York. (1987). *Home care in New York City: Providers, payers, and clients.* New York, N.Y.

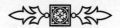

# CHAPTER

# Administrative Operational Requirements

Susan Craig Schulmerich

The administration of a home health agency is similar to the administration of any health care delivery program. There are

- operational and patient care regulations on the federal, state, local, quasi-public, and payer level. Payers in general do not have their own "conditions of participation" but defer to the federal, state, and quasi-public conditions.
- industry standards and practices
- professional practice standards

However, home care seems to have more than its share of burdensome, conflicting, and repetitive regulations and requirements. Perhaps this results from the vastness of the care delivery sites, the lack of immediate on-site supervision of care delivery personnel, or the perceived opportunity for fraud. Whatever the reason, compliance efforts are costly, not only financially, but in administrative and care giver time. For example, at the 1990 Legislative and Regulatory Conference in Washington, D.C., sponsored by the National Association for Home Care, it was reported that 30 to 50 percent of a professional care giver's time was spent completing mandated paperwork. At the same conference, a participant produced the *average* package of paper necessary to submit a $30,000 home care claim—272 pieces of paper. Conversely, a hospital submits two forms for a claim, a *universal billing form* and a *physician attestation,* no matter what the dollar amount. This chapter will review the basic aspects of regulatory requirements as they affect payment streams, the governing authority of an agency, and required committees in an agency.

# CUSTOMARY REGULATION OF AN AGENCY

Regardless of the type of agency, there are federal regulatory requirements for *certified home health agencies* (CHHAs) and Medicare (M/C) certified hospice programs. At a minimum, most states have some form of licensure for CHHAs as well as other non-M/C home health organizations.

## State Regulations

Each state has peculiar and unique regulations. A discussion of individual state subtleties is far beyond the scope of this work. Readers are directed to investigate the state regulations where they practice.

However, with that said, an example of what faces an agency in meeting various state regulatory requirements will illustrate the most common day-to-day difficulties of dealing with bureaucracies.

On a state level, New York is recognized as having the most burdensome regulations of any state in the union. As mentioned earlier, the upper range of time spent by professional care givers completing paperwork was most assuredly in New York State. Within the state bureaucracies, various departments, such as the health department, social service, and human resource administration, may all write regulations affecting the delivery of home care service. Unfortunately for the patients and providers, there may be little to no dialogue between the departments. The result is conflicting regulations that home care providers either work through, work around, or initiate legal action to have the regulations enjoined.

An example will illustrate the problem. In New York State, the Department of Health (DoH) writes and enforces the regulations; the Department of Social Service (DSS) pays for the care. In 1993, DSS announced a cost containment initiative that would result in the reduction of home health aide hours paid for by the department. The core of this initiative was to place patients who had very high utilization of home health aide hours in a less expensive alternate delivery system. If a *patient* were to refuse placement, DSS would stop all payment to the agency. When agencies inquired as to who would pay for the services, the answer was, ". . . not DSS." DoH regulations prohibit discharging a patient for loss of or lack of payment source. When representatives of both departments were brought together with providers, there was no resolution of the uncompensated care issue. Providers had no alternative but to seek an injunction through the courts to stop DSS from implementing its cost containment plan. At the end of 1994, the issue had still not been settled.

Since each state is unique, regulatory requirements will focus on federal *conditions of participation* (COPs) and the quasi-public accrediting bodies, Joint Commission on Accreditation of Healthcare Organizations (JCAHO) and the Community Health Accreditation Program (CHAP).

# THE FEDERAL GOVERNMENT

When M/C and Medicaid (M/A) were legislated in 1965, the federal government needed an organization that would be responsible for administering the immense new programs. The Health Care Financing Administration (HCFA) is that organization. It is responsible for promulgating the COPs and overseeing the compliance with those conditions.

Congress enacts M/C and M/A legislation and then sends it to HCFA to develop and write the regulatory language. Regulatory language subsequently becomes the COPs. For an agency to be eligible for M/C direct reimbursement, it must adhere to standards of care and administrative processes that HCFA considers to be the minimum level to justify the expenditure of M/C tax dollars.

Among other things, the COPs address

- patient care
- administration of an agency
- patient rights and responsibilities
- quality management programs

Conformity with the COPs is supposed to be reviewed and evaluated by HCFA on an annual basis. In order to meet this requirement, HCFA can assign responsibility to conduct compliance surveys to appropriate state offices or departments. The achievement record of various states in meeting the annual survey process, and the *consistent* interpretation of the COPs, has not been uniform. In an effort to correct inconsistencies, HCFA granted *deemed status* to JCAHO and CHAP in 1993. *Deemed status* means that an organization is acting in the place of HCFA for evaluation of compliance to COPs. If an agency is accredited by either JCAHO or CHAP, then the federal COPs are considered to have been met for the year in which the survey took place, thus obviating the need for a state agency to conduct a survey.

## JCAHO and CHAP

Accreditation by either JCAHO or CHAP indicates the agency has met a minimum standard for patient care and operational administration. With increasing frequency, managed care organizations, in their *requests for proposal,* require accreditation in order to even give *consideration* to applicants; provider status almost always necessitates accreditation. Also, CHHAs that subcontract for services such as home medical equipment (HME), infusion, or home health aide service are requiring accreditation as a condition for contract award.

Should an agency choose to have JCAHO or CHAP conduct the survey for COPs compliance, the survey must

- be unannounced
- take place every year

It does *not* automatically relieve the agency from survey by the state health department.

If a state's regulations are more stringent than the federal COPs, or the state laws do not permit abdication of responsibility to another organization, the state agency responsible for licensure would have to conduct its own survey on whatever schedule the law requires. If an agency declines deemed status from one of the accrediting organizations, then the surveyors will be *invited* to evaluate the agency on a triennial schedule.

## Deficiencies

If an agency is unable to fulfill the COPs and/or the state requirements, a number of unpleasant sanctions can be enforced. For instance, fines can be levied, contracted management can be put in place, acceptance of new cases can be suspended, or operations can be discontinued all together.

Fortunately there are appeal mechanisms. However, they are costly from a legal and revenue standpoint. Also, the reputation of the agency may be irreparably damaged. The accrediting organizations, whether public or quasi-public, do not impose severe sanctions unless the operation of the agency presents a real and present danger to the public.

An administrator of a home care agency is well-advised to stay informed of the federal, state, payer, and accrediting body rules, regulations, and standards in order to avoid the consequences of noncompliance. Also to be considered are the issues of fraud and abuse, antitrust, and the practice of exclusivity, which can be perpetrated by unprincipled and unethical individuals and organizations. Without a doubt, there is a place and need for regulation and survey, providing the rules and processes are uniform, consistently applied, and not redundant.

# GOVERNING BODY

The governing body of an agency may also be known as the Board of Trustees or the Board of Directors. Irrespective of the title, the governing body is vested with the overall authority and responsibility for operation of the agency, which includes

- general management
- fiscal accountability
- quality management
- compliance with federal, state, and local laws regarding equal opportunity, nondiscrimination, conflict of interest, and so forth

When reviewing the obligations of the governing body, using either accreditation standards or state regulations, it becomes evident that this is an awesome responsibility, not to be taken lightly. The governing body usually relinquishes day-to-day agency operation to an administrator who assumes the responsibility and authority of the governing body.

## Composition of the Governing Body

Depending on the status of the agency—freestanding, hospital-based, public, or charitable—the governing body will vary in structure. For instance, in a hospital-based agency the governing body may be a subcommittee of the hospital Board of Trustees. In a charitable organization, it might be members of the clergy that make up the governing body; in the public sector it may be members of the community where the agency operates. Notwithstanding the composition, the responsibilities are the same—total accountability for the operation and actions of the organization. Because of this serious responsibility, accrediting organizations are making orientation of all incumbent and future members of the governing authority a requirement.

### *Quality Management Responsibilities*

Gaining more attention, from accrediting bodies in particular, is the accountability of the governing authority for the total quality management (TQM) and continuous quality improvement (CQI) program of the agency. The governing authority is an active participant in the TQM/CQI program and will be more so in the future. At the scheduled meetings of the governing body, a portion of the agenda must be devoted to TQM/CQI activities and program planning. During survey interviews with the governing body, it can be expected that the surveyor will ascertain the knowledge and involvement of the members of the governing body in the TQM/CQI program.

# PROFESSIONAL ADVISORY GROUPS

An organization cannot rely solely on its own internal resources to identify areas of opportunity for improvement, expanded practice, and enhancement of program scope. Therefore, outside resources are utilized through a systematic process of committee development such as *professional advisory committee, utilization review,* and *physician advisory.* The functions and responsibilities of these committees are specific to, and based upon, regulatory requirements and operational needs. The generic function of the committee is more important than the name of the committee.

## Professional Advisory Committee

A professional advisory committee is designed to assist agency management in identifying program needs and enhancements as recommended by referral sources and consumers. Obviously, with this purpose in mind, there is a significant focus on TQM/CQI.

The membership of the committee should be represented by

- referral sources
- consumers
- contractors the agency conducts business with
- professional disciplines from the agency
- administrative staff

## Utilization Review

This committee is charged with analyzing a representative sample of patients cared for during a particular period of time. A representative sample is generally a percentage of the expected total average daily census (ADC) for the year. If the ADC is expected to be 500 patients, then 10 percent, or fifty cases, will be reviewed during the calendar year. If the committee meets on a quarterly basis, 12 to 13 records are reviewed during the meeting. The focus of the analysis is usually on

- appropriateness of service provided
- timeliness of service
- rendering of services actually ordered
- that there was justifiable reason(s) for cases not accepted for service
- what percentage of the patients reach the goals developed at the time of admission

Additionally, this committee reviews all patient incidents or occurrences for the period being analyzed.

## Physician Advisory Committee

Since the direct patient care staff of the agency is practicing in an "unsupervised" environment, and the availability of immediate consultation in the event of an emergency is not always possible, the physician advisory committee develops a set of policies, or standing orders, for the professional staff in the event of an emergency. This committee also develops medical relationship policies, and procedures to follow for physician-related issues.

These are just a sampling of committees and their respective responsibilities necessary to operate a home care agency. Each agency creates committees that meet the operational needs of the organization and address the requirements of regulatory authorities.

## CONCLUSION

The administrative responsibilities associated with the operation of a home health agency are expansive and require the attention of any number of administrative staff. However, it is the ultimate responsibility of the governing authority to ensure that the administration of the agency and the standing committees are effective in their respective charges and contribute positively to the TQM/CQI effort.

## *Suggested Readings*

Joint Commission on Accreditation of Healthcare Organizations. (1994). *Accreditation Manual 1995.* Chicago: JCAHO.

Rooney, A.L. & Vavrinchik, D. (1993). JCAHO standards and quality management. *Hospital home care strategic management for integrated care delivery.* Chicago: American Hospital Association.

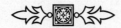

# CHAPTER

# Administrative Structure

**Susan Craig Schulmerich**

The administrative organization of an agency depends upon a number of things.

- Is the agency freestanding, part of a chain, a department within a hospital, or a public agency?
- Is the agency certified or licensed?
- Is there one office or a main office with multiple satellites?
- Is the agency licensed in more than one state?
- What is the annual visit volume?
- What is the scope of service provided by the agency?
- Is the agency in a rural or urban area?
- Is the agency unionized; and what categories of staff are affected?

All these questions have a bearing on the administrative structure, but the last four—size, scope, geographic location, and unionization—have the most profound effect and will be the focus of this discussion.

Although agency types differ, there are common position titles, functions, and personnel requirements. Such similarities will be addressed in this section as well.

# AGENCY SIZE

Agency size has the single greatest impact on the administrative structure, irrespective of the agency type (freestanding, hospital-based, and so on). For obvious reasons, an agency that performs 25,000 visits a *year* versus one that makes 25,000 visits a *month* will have remarkably different tables of organization, as well as just about everything else! Agency size affects the number and types of departments and the functional responsibilities of those departments. The visit volume, which is the same as size, dictates the number of field staff required to make visits. The number of support staff such as payroll, personnel, clerical, and escort/drivers is dictated by the number of field staff. The number of field staff and support staff dictates the number of administrative staff necessary to supervisor agency activities. The entire structure is symbiotic.

# SCOPE OF SERVICE

In Medicare (M/C) certified agencies, at least one qualifying service (skilled nursing, physical therapy, or speech therapy) must be provided by staff who are employees of the agency. Proposed federal regulations will require that 67 percent of service must be provided by employees of the agency. This will have a chilling effect on the number of *independent* contractors who currently provide service to agencies. The use of independent contractors has lessened in the recent past as a result of IRS scrutiny into the position status of these professionals. If independent contractors do not pass the litmus test of autonomous practice and self direction, their status will change from independent to employee.

The broader the scope of service an agency provides, the larger and more diverse the staff required to perform the service. For example, if an agency has truly "one-stop shopping," the complexity and number of staff necessary to operate the "home care supermarket" escalate proportionately. Personnel savings are found more through efficiency initiatives, such as automation, rather than economy of scale. The reason for this is simple; as visit volume grows, the direct care staff necessary to see the increased patient volume can only be accomplished in two ways—adding direct care staff, or reducing or eliminating non-patient activities such as paperwork. And, as stated earlier, the larger the direct care roster, the greater the number of staff needed to support them.

The staffing of a home care agency can be compared to a military model in that the troops (direct care staff) need to be supported by a variety of services. These services include quartermaster (general stores and supplies), a motor pool (vehicles), officers (administrative staff), and so on. The ratio of staff required to support the direct care givers can be as high as one-to-one, depending on the nuances of the state in which the agency is located. It is well-known by providers, and acknowledged in the industry, that home care is *paper intense*. Paper documentation has to be sorted, processed, filed, stored, and otherwise manipulated to assure availability for inspection and review by any number of organizations and agencies. Administrative overhead for clerical and support functions can be an appreciable cost to an agency. As the industry moves toward a health care *information highway* the manipulation of paper will be reduced, but there will always be a need for support personnel to manage data. Professional field staff productivity and supervisor staff ratios will be discussed in Chapter 18.

# GEOGRAPHIC LOCATION

No matter what the location of the agency is, whether in a sprawling rural area or the inner city, each type of location uniquely influences the number of personnel needed. Direct care staff working in a rural area may have incredible distances to travel between visits and to and from the office. If this is the case, the expected productivity in a rural agency would be less than the productivity of a nurse who has a daily caseload in one square city block. Also, the actual patient visit time is probably higher in the rural setting, in comparison to an inner city resident, simply because the patient may have restricted access to health care providers. It can be expected that limited or restricted access to providers, other than the agency staff, will extend assessment, evaluation, and treatment times. Reduced visit productivity inflates the number of direct care staff needed to manage the patient volume.

Unfortunately, urban agencies are faced with problems such as street crime, drug trafficking, domestic violence, and street gangs. The need to protect the field staff becomes a priority for agency management (see Chapter 22 for security issues). Protection takes the form of escort/drivers, agency automobiles, and cellular phones, to name a few. Not only do these "protective" personnel and equipment have an immediate cost, but they require oversight and routine replacement. If inner cities continue to deteriorate, the areas necessitating protection will expand and the issues of staff safety will intensify, adding to the number of personnel needed and the costs of providing care.

# UNIONIZATION

The traditional union environment, an adversarial relationship between management and labor, can have a negative impact on morale, teamwork, collaboration, and the economic affairs of the organization. Fortunately, the tide is changing. Labor and management recognize the health of the organization is a dual responsibility; both parties share, perhaps not equally, but nonetheless share, responsibility.

However, even in the new enlightened atmosphere of labor relations, unionization forces issues of supervision, division of labor, and protectionism to the forefront of agency organization. When an agency cannot make rapid changes in the work environment to take innovative and sometimes defensive action or capitalize on a new business opportunity, it can find itself at a serious market disadvantage. Investments in modern technology to improve productivity, reduce overtime, enhance employee efficiency, and ultimately be able to do more with the same number of staff, are generally in opposition to union objectives. Management must cultivate an environment of trust with labor unions, as described in Chapter 7, in order to accomplish its goals of maintaining a competitive edge in the market place.

# FUNCTIONAL DEPARTMENTS

The configuration of *any* home health agency will have similarities. The differences that exist are a result of size, scope of service, ownership, and state idiosyncracies. Similarities and generic functions will be reviewed in this chapter.

## Administration

Agency administration is responsible for

- day-to-day operations
- short- and long-term planning
- budget development and oversight
- compliance with federal, state, and quasi-public regulating authorities
- development of policy and procedures characteristic to the organization

How the administration accomplishes these charges depends on the variables mentioned earlier—size, scope, ownership, and regulation.

### Size and Ownership

Division of departments and functions of those departments are directly affected by the size and ownership of an agency. In Chapter 9, financial tables of organization for agencies with differing sizes and ownership are illustrated. These tables demonstrate the complexity of an organization based on the two variables.

If an agency has a modest visit volume and is part of a department of a hospital, *hospital-related* organization, a chain, or one of several satellites, it may utilize the departments and services of the parent or primary organization for operational elements such as

- personnel
- legal and risk management
- occupational health service
- finance, home health finance is *significantly* different from hospital finance. The finance section (Section II) discusses the obvious and not so obvious differences. Relying on the finance department of the hospital may not be the best strategy for a hospital-related agency. (*Hospital-related* is a term used to describe a home health agency that has a direct relationship with a hospital, or hospitals, but is not a department of the hospital(s). For example, the governing body of the agency may be comprised of representatives of any number of competing hospitals whose common tie is the home health agency.)
- real estate, building, and maintenance service
- management information systems
- general stores, and so forth

If, on the other hand, the agency has an appreciable patient volume, requires space apart from the main affiliation, and has a large work force, it may act and be treated more like a freestanding agency. The agency may rely very little on, or receive limited support from, the parent organization. If this is the case, the administrative structure of the agency will mirror or perhaps duplicate the parent organization.

## Scope of Service

An agency that provides a broad array of care and service through its own staff and unique programs, such as infusion, home medical equipment (HME), and home health aides, will have a correspondingly greater number of staff employed than an agency that subcontracts for particular patient care services and programmatic needs. Although this seems obvious, the complexity of the tables of organization and lines of communication showing administrative structure sometimes need the service of a cartographer to decipher. As reported at *Competitive Strategies for Home Care* (1994), a conference held in California, the largest freestanding agency in the United States is *Visiting Nurse Service of New York* (VNSNY). The table of organization for the provision of 1.5 million professional visits annually along with paraprofessional visits of 13 million hours has an administrative and program structure that is incomprehensible without a guide! Multi-hospital home health agencies have equally confusing tables of organization, as do single hospital-based agencies that may be part of an academic teaching facility.

## State Idiosyncracies

Individual states run the spectrum of standards, from rigid control and mandates, such as New York, to rather relaxed state standards. The subtleties of each state are well beyond the extent of this book and the reader is referred to individual state codes and regulation.

However, with that said, state regulations can have an enormous impact on required administrative and nondirect care giving staff. Additionally, emerging federal regulations for Occupational Health and Safety Administration (OSHA) blood-borne pathogen guidelines, equal opportunity laws, and so forth, require human resources to assure compliance with the directives. Public policy increases the number *and* types of nonclinical staff required to continue the operation of the agency.

### Quasi-Public Organizations

Joint Commission on Accreditation of Health Care Organizations (JCAHO) and Community Health Accreditation Program (CHAP) require specific position functions to be part of the table of organization. For example, both accrediting programs require a governing authority, an administrator, and a clinical director. In the 1995 standards for JCAHO there is a requirement for an accountable person for information management (1994). What additional changes will be required by health care reform is open to speculation. However, with a high degree of certainty there will have to be at least one department that oversees the administration of managed care and capitated contracts.

# POSITION TITLES AND FUNCTIONS

Each agency will identify positions required to achieve regulatory compliance and operational needs. As has been previously identified, there are commonalities across all types of agencies. The function of certain jobs, irrespective of the title, is yet another commonality. Clinical position titles and functions can be found in Chapter 20. Financial titles and functions, as mentioned earlier, can be found in Chapter 9. Administrative, nonclinical staff will be covered here.

Educational preparation, other than education required for professional licensure and that required by regulating authorities, is an important aspect of position qualifications. Minimally, administrative staff should hold an undergraduate degree in a position-related discipline. A graduate degree in the appropriate "specialty" would be advantageous. However, germane and verifiable experience can and should be considered when a candidate is evaluated for an administrative position if the educational credentials are weak.

## Administrator

The generic title of administrator describes the person responsible to the governing body for the management of the agency. Previous home care experience is not a hard and fast requirement for the position, nor is clinical licensure, but one or both certainly helps. What is required is a person who

- is able to effect change with the least amount of trauma
- enjoys an ever-changing work environment
- is able to anticipate change
- sees change as an opportunity

In other words, an administrator is a *change agent.* In order for the administrator to be the agent of change, (s)he must be able to delegate *and* empower the management and other staff to implement change. Empowering the work force is discussed in Chapter 7.

The customary titles of the administrator are

• Executive Director
• Chief Executive Officer
• President
• Administrative Director
• Director

## Clinical Director

There must be a person responsible and accountable for the clinical services provided by the agency. Clinical services, skilled nursing, physical therapy, and so forth, provided directly by the agency, and subcontracted services such as paraprofessional care, infusion, and HME are under the direction and oversight of the clinical director.

The federal conditions of participation (COPs) place the responsibility for patient care coordination on the certified home health agency (CHHA). In turn, the governing body, through the director of the agency, holds the clinical director accountable for the quality of care delivered by *all* providers. Irrespective of agency size, in order for the clinical director to fulfill the impressive obligations of the position, first- and second-line clinical managers will most certainly be required.

Unlike the administrator, this position requires a licensed professional who has extensive experience in home care. The clinical director must understand the function and responsibilities of the other professional disciplines, as well as the role of the various subcontract organizations.

The titles customarily assigned to this important position are

• Chief Clinical Officer
• Director of Patient Services
• Vice President of Patient Services
• Clinical Manager

## Director of Administrative Services

The Director of Administrative Services is the equivalent of a Chief Operating Officer in a hospital setting and is responsible for nonclinical operations. Nonclinical departments include payroll, personnel, building maintenance, purchasing, medical records, and so forth. Depending on agency size, the Director of Administrative Services may also be responsible for the financial functions of the business.

The qualifications for this position are similar to the Director—an experienced manager with a comprehensive background in directing multiple, functionally dissimilar departments.

Other descriptive titles for this position are

- Chief Operating Officer
- Director of Support Services
- Director of Nonclinical Services
- Business Manager

## Director of Information Services

The home care industry is moving at "warp" speed toward fully integrated information systems. While many agencies have not reached the point of either fashioning an *information systems (IS) department* or creating a position of Director of IS, the time is rapidly approaching that both will be a necessity. With the advent of managed care and capitation, IS is the *only* way an agency will be able to coordinate the variety of benefit plans and payor stipulations that will be a result of the new health care reimbursement environment. The 1995 JCAHO standards devote an entire section to *information management.*

The qualifications for the position will depend a great deal on whether the department already exists or if it is a "start-up" operation. At a minimum, an undergraduate degree in computer science, and experience as second in command of an IS department or as clinical information system project manager should be required.

Other titles descriptive of this position are

- Chief Information Officer
- Director of Management Information Services

## Chief Financial Officer

This position and its responsibilities and qualifications are described in detail in Chapter 9. The importance of the Chief Financial Officer *cannot* be understated. Home care reimbursement and finance are so intricate, different, and confusing that one person should be responsible for managing the financial aspects of the agency.

Other titles for this position include

- Director of Finance
- Director of Reimbursement
- Vice President of Finance

## Other Positions

If an agency is in an expansion phase, perhaps purchasing and implementing capital projects, developing new clinical programs, acquiring existing businesses, "re-engineering" operations, opening new offices, or possibly engaging in several of these simultaneously, it would be wise to consider having one person responsible for the overall direction of the activities, such as a *Director of Special Projects.* In the business of home care there is *always* a special project on the horizon. Once the special project is completed or implemented and requires ongoing administration, it can be assigned to one of the operations management staff.

An agency needs the consultative service of a *Medical Director.* There are many areas a medical director should be involved in, such as

- developing medical relationship policies
- conducting meetings of the physician advisory council
- intervening with referring physicians in the event of a conflict with professional staff
- participating in patient-centered case conferences
- participating in quality management activities

The number of full-time equivalent (FTE) first and second line managers and non-management staff necessary to accomplish the responsibilities of the senior management titles will differ from agency to agency. Unfortunately there is no "cookbook" ratio of management to nonmanagement FTEs. Sometimes management staffing requirements are developed through "gut instinct." Other times, management engineers are consulted. And other times, *history* is the force that dictates management positions.

## CONCLUSION

The organization and administration of a home health agency is far more complex and complicated than many health care professionals and administrators understand. The number of staff required to provide care and administer the program is directly affected by four primary elements

- size (visit volume)
- scope of service
- geographic location
- unionization

## REFERENCE

*Competitive Strategies for Home Care Providers.* (1994). Conference held in San Diego, CA; September 22–23, 1994.

## *Suggested Reading*

Gilliland, J.C. (1993). Employment issues and personnel policies. *Hospital home care strategic management for integrated care delivery.* Chicago: American Hospital Association.

Gilliland, J.C. (1993). Employment issues such as independent contractors, employment applications, overtime, and minimum wage. *Hospital home care strategic management for integrated care delivery.* Chicago: American Hospital Association.

Joint Commission on Accreditation of Healthcare Organizations. (1994). *1995 Accreditation Manual for Home Health Care.* Oakbrook, IL: JCAHO.

# CHAPTER

# Total Quality Management and Its Relationship to Marketing

Susan Craig Schulmerich

It may seem odd to incorporate *total quality management* (TQM) with marketing for a chapter topic. However, the health care reimbursement environment is rapidly moving toward the methodology of *outcome measurements* to determine the appropriateness of an agency to be a provider to managed care organizations (MCOs). Traditionally, physicians, hospitals, nursing homes, and community groups were the primary marketing targets of home care. Today the marketing focus is to payers—networks, alliances, health maintenance organizations (HMOs), preferred provider organizations (PPOs), and so forth.

The federal government, Joint Commission on Accreditation of Health Care Organizations (JCAHO), and Community Health Accreditation Program (CHAP) are directing their respective regulatory and survey focuses on outcome measures. Compliance with the federal conditions of participation (COPs) and accreditation by either JCAHO or CHAP will be a requirement of many, if not all, payers in the near future. Marketing endeavors of an agency will have to be supported by measurable, objective data indicating the value, worth, and contribution of the agency's interventions in relation to the patients' positive experiences. Regulatory compliance and all associated documentation requirements are challenging to agency operations. Substantial noncompliance with any of the regulatory bodies jeopardizes the viability of an agency, and correction of weaknesses or deficiencies can be painfully expensive. A fully-integrated quality management program is the appropriate venue to monitor and identify regulatory compliance issues *before* they become problems.

Abundant resources on TQM and continuous quality improvement (CQI) are available. It is not the purpose of this chapter to condense the resources. Rather, outcome measures, how to incorporate them into the agency TQM/CQI program, and how to use them in marketing and setting contract parameters will be discussed.

# ORGANIZATION OF QUALITY MANAGEMENT

Whatever the size of an agency, there must be one person directing a discrete department responsible for the TQM/CQI program and plan. Obviously, the size and activity of the agency will dictate how large the department will be and what monetary resources will be budgeted. Operationally, there must be *one* person whose function is to coordinate and guide the program. However, as will be discussed in *Empowering Employees for Excellence, Energy, and Enthusiasm* (Chapter 7), the most senior-ranking person in the organization is ultimately responsible and must take an active part in the TQM/CQI program.

## Regulatory Compliance

The myriad of regulations promulgated by various levels of government and quasi-public organizations are astounding. Compliance with the regulations, and monitoring that compliance, requires diligent attention by one person and/or department.

Therefore, a natural correlation exists between regulatory compliance and TQM/CQI. The agency program should incorporate regulatory requirements as part of the overall TQM plan. In this way the TQM/CQI director and department become accountable for activities associated with federal COPs, state licensure, local regulations, and accreditation requirements. Later in this chapter, in *The TQM/CQI Department*, regulatory compliance monitoring will be discussed.

## The Director of TQM/CQI

In the organizational table of an agency, the person responsible for the TQM/CQI program must have a title, position, and authority within the structure that allows autonomy, self direction, and accountability. In most instances, the position is one of staff rather than line responsibility. However, in larger agencies, depending on the diversity of responsibilities, the administrator for TQM/CQI may have line responsibility as well.

The administration for TQM/CQI requires a person who is thoroughly familiar with the theories and concepts of quality management and, most importantly, is able to effectively communicate this familiarity both orally and in writing. Additionally, the person must have comprehensive knowledge of the regulations and standards for home care. In other words, this is not a position that encourages "on the job training." The person must come to the post with an extensive understanding of

1. quality management in home care
2. standards of a variety of professional practice groups
3. standards of accrediting bodies
4. federal regulations

A seasoned clinician with skills in

- communicating (written and verbal)
- teaching
- analytical problem solving
- team building
- creating an energized environment

is just the person for the job!

# THE TQM/CQI DEPARTMENT

The department requires human and information management resources to fulfill its responsibilities. In the 1995 JCAHO standards for home care, the attention to TQM/CQI is most impressive, and vastly expands previous standards. In order to meet the TQM/CQI requirements, there must be a dedicated person and department with all *resources necessary* to achieve the quality management plan. The standards specifically address the role and responsibilities of the governing authority in committing the resources to accomplish the annual goals and objectives of the TQM/CQI program. On a regular and scheduled basis, the governing authority must be made aware of the department's progress toward the stated goals, and an appraisal must be made.

## The Responsibilities of the TQM/CQI Department

It may seem absurd to detail the responsibilities of the department. Its very title indicates the obligation it has to the overall organization. But, a well-defined, tightly organized TQM/CQI section has many more responsibilities than are evident and assumed.

### Regulatory Compliance and Associated Documentation

Again, because of the variety of state, city, and local regulations, which are literally impossible to cover in any text, only federal regulations and accrediting body standards will be dealt with in this section.

*The 485.* For a patient to be cared for, there must be a physician's *plan of care* (POC). For Medicare (M/C) the POC is written on a 485, a Health Care Financing Administration (HCFA) form detailing, among other things

- the services needed, why they are needed, and for how long
- the medications a patient is receiving
- equipment needed
- living arrangements, which is defined as whether the patient lives alone, with a spouse, family member(s), or another person, or has a support system within the community in which he or she lives
- prognosis

Demographic information is also gleaned from the 485. In the COPs, HCFA stipulates that a signed 485 must be on the patient record within fourteen days of admission to the home care program. Figure 5.1 is a HCFA 485.

Obtaining signed 485s is not as simple as it may seem. In many instances the POC is not developed until the patient has been discharged from the hospital. The *Clinical Section* (Section III beginning with chapter seven) provides general clinical management process, concerns, and issues. The entire procedure for creating, generating, mailing, receiving, and recording a 485 is one of the appropriate functions of the TQM department. The department's success at mastering just this process is worth the costs associated with operating the program. Without the POC an agency cannot bill (M/C) for service provided. For that matter, an agency cannot bill any payer for services unless the services have been ordered by a physician. Also, without a physician-signed POC the agency could be accused of practicing medicine without a license.

The importance of the POC is obvious, and the liabilities for not complying with the law can be distressing. A primary objective of any TQM/CQI program is to reduce risk. Tracking and following up on POCs is a focused activity for the reduction of risk and the assurance of financial health for the agency.

***The 487.***   During any admission to a home care program, changes in the POC can be expected. The 487 is HCFA's answer to modifications in the original plan as it appeared on the 485. Figure 5.2 is a sample of a 487. The 487s need to be generated, mailed, tracked, and recorded just as 485s do. Again, this is a natural activity for the quality management department.

***The 486 and 488.***   The reader may wonder why there is separation of HCFA form numbers; why are they not in succession? The 486 is the end of the first-month summary of the current certification period of care. The *certification period* is a two-month or sixty-two-day time frame for the care of a patient. At the end of this time period, if the patient requires continued care, a *recertification* is requested. The recertification is for an additional two months or sixty-two days, and is processed in the same manner as a certification. At one time a 486 was required with each 485 in order to submit the claim to the fiscal intermediary (FI) for payment. The fiscal intermediary is the organization under contract with HCFA to process and pay claims for M/C covered services. In 1992, HCFA pardoned agencies from routinely submitting 486s and now requires a 486 only if a 488 is generated by the FI. A 488 is a *request to develop* a claim. If the FI has a problem interpreting a submitted claim, or is conducting a specific type of review on a population of particular diagnoses, then the 488 will be initiated. Figures 5.3 and 5.4 are samples of a 486 and 488, respectively.

It should be clear that the paperwork associated with regulatory compliance not only requires a department to deal with it, but regulatory paperwork is a critical quality, risk, and financial management issue.

# PATIENT OUTCOMES

The effectiveness of care provided to patients has become the focal point of nearly every payer and regulating organization. One challenge that faces the home care industry is that there is little to no *benchmarking* data from which to determine "how good is good" or how ABC Agency compares, with XYZ Agency.

## Absence of Universal Definitions

Part of the perplexing issue of benchmarking stems from the lack of an industry-generated universal data set (definitions) of what home care is and what components constitute a home care organization. In 1993, the National Association for Home Care (NAHC) enlisted public and private sector home health care representatives from all geographic areas to define the various parameters, tasks, and operational terminology associated with the industry, excluding HME and infusion services. The Universal Data Set Task Force was able to reach consensus on approximately 75 percent of the terms needing definition. The remaining 25 percent continue to be crafted in order to find common ground from which to gain consensus. The lack of universal terms and

# HOME HEALTH CERTIFICATION AND PLAN OF CARE

| 1. Patient's HI Claim No. | 2. Start Of Care Date | 3. Certification Period | | 4. Medical Record No. | 5. Provider No. |
|---|---|---|---|---|---|
| | | From: | To: | | |

**6. Patient's Name and Address**

**7. Provider's Name, Address and Telephone Number**

| 8. Date of Birth | 9. Sex ☐ M ☐ F |
|---|---|

**10. Medications: Dose/Frequency/Route (N)ew (C)hanged**

| 11. ICD-9-CM | Principal Diagnosis | Date |
|---|---|---|

| 12. ICD-9-CM | Surgical Procedure | Date |
|---|---|---|

| 13. ICD-9-CM | Other Pertinent Diagnoses | Date |
|---|---|---|

**14. DME and Supplies**

**15. Safety Measures:**

**16. Nutritional Req.**

**17. Allergies:**

**18.A. Functional Limitations**

| 1 ☐ Amputation | 5 ☐ Paralysis | 9 ☐ Legally Blind |
| 2 ☐ Bowel/Bladder (Incontinence) | 6 ☐ Endurance | A ☐ Dyspnea With Minimal Exertion |
| 3 ☐ Contracture | 7 ☐ Ambulation | B ☐ Other (Specify) |
| 4 ☐ Hearing | 8 ☐ Speech | |

**18.B. Activities Permitted**

| 1 ☐ Complete Bedrest | 6 ☐ Partial Weight Bearing | A ☐ Wheelchair |
| 2 ☐ Bedrest BRP | 7 ☐ Independent At Home | B ☐ Walker |
| 3 ☐ Up As Tolerated | 8 ☐ Crutches | C ☐ No Restrictions |
| 4 ☐ Transfer Bed/Chair | 9 ☐ Cane | D ☐ Other (Specify) |
| 5 ☐ Exercises Prescribed | | |

**19. Mental Status:**

| 1 ☐ Oriented | 3 ☐ Forgetful | 5 ☐ Disoriented | 7 ☐ Agitated |
| 2 ☐ Comatose | 4 ☐ Depressed | 6 ☐ Lethargic | 8 ☐ Other |

**20. Prognosis:**

| 1 ☐ Poor | 2 ☐ Guarded | 3 ☐ Fair | 4 ☐ Good | 5 ☐ Excellent |

21. Orders for Discipline and Treatments (Specify Amount/Frequency/Duration)

22. Goals/Rehabilitation Potential/Discharge Plans

23. Nurse's Signature and Date of Verbal SOC Where Applicable:

25. Date HHA Received Signed POT

24. Physician's Name and Address

26. I certify/recertify that this patient is confined to his/her home and needs intermittent skilled nursing care, physical therapy and/or speech therapy or continues to need occupational therapy. The patient is under my care, and I have authorized the services on this plan of care and will periodically review the plan.

27. Attending Physician's Signature and Date Signed

28. Anyone who misrepresents, falsifies, or conceals essential information required for payment of Federal funds may be subject to fine, imprisonment, or civil penalty under applicable Federal laws.

PROVIDER

Form HCFA-485 (C-4) (02-94)

**FIGURE 5.1**

Department of Health and Human Services
Health Care Financing Administration

Form Approved
OMB No. 0938-0357

**ADDENDUM TO:** ☐ **PLAN OF TREATMENT** ☐ **MEDICAL UPDATE**

| 1. Patient's HI Claim No. | 2. SOC Date | 3. Certification Period | 4. Medical Record No. | 5. Provider No. |
|---|---|---|---|---|
| | | From:          To: | | |

6. Patient's Name

7. Provider Name

8. Item
No.

| 9. Signature of Physician | 10. Date |
| 11. Optional Name/Signature of Nurse/Therapist | 12. Date |

**PROVIDER**

Form HCFA-487 (C4) (4-87)

**FIGURE 5.2**

# MEDICAL UPDATE AND PATIENT INFORMATION

| 1. Patient's HI Claim No. | 2. SOC Date | 3. Certification Period | 4. Medical Record No. | 5. Provider No. |
|---|---|---|---|---|
| | | From:    To: | | |

6. Patient's Name and Address

7. Provider's Name

8. Medicare Covered: ☐ Y   ☐ N

9. Date Physician Last Saw Patient:

10. Date Last Contacted Physician:

11. Is the Patient Receiving Care in an 1861 (J)(1) Skilled Nursing Facility or Equivalent?   ☐ Y   ☐ N   ☐ Do Not Know

12.   ☐ Certification   ☐ Recertification   ☐ Modified

13. Dates of Last Inpatient Stay: Admission     Discharge

14. Type of Facility:

15. Updated information: New Orders/Treatments/Clinical Facts/Summary from Each Discipline

16. Functional Limitations (Expand From 485 and Level of ADL) Reason Homebound/Prior Functional Status

17. Supplementary Plan of Care on File from Physician Other than Referring Physician:
(If Yes, Please Specify Giving Goals/Rehab. Potential/Discharge Plan)

☐ Y  ☐ N

18. Unusual Home/Social Environment

19. Indicate Any Time When the Home Health Agency Made a Visit and Patient was Not Home and Reason Why if Ascertainable

20. Specify Any Known Medical and/or Non-Medical Reasons the Patient Regularly Leaves Home and Frequency of Occurrence

21. Nurse or Therapist Completing or Reviewing Form

Date (Mo., Day, Yr.)

**PROVIDER**

Form HCFA-486 (C3) (02-94)

**FIGURE 5.3**

# UNITED
# GOVERNMENT
# SERVICES

▼

## HOME HEALTH AGENCY INTERMEDIARY MEDICAL INFORMATION REQUEST
(Computer generated 488 form)

IRC/03a
Request Date: 03/15/94

Provider No:                               Patient:
    HOSP HM CAR                     HICN:
                         DCN: 0594070832400-P

To process your claim, the information listed below is needed by Medical
Review. This information must be received by Medicare Medical Review
by the 40th calendar day from the request date or the claim will be sent to
the LIMO file.

Please submit the following information for Home Health services of
01-12-94 through 01-31-94 for beneficiary with medical record number of
:

—All applicable physician signed plans of care (485, 486, and 487);

—All signed physician orders pertaining to the plan(s) of care.

Return this form as a cover sheet for identification of requested information.
Mail requested information to:

ATTN: Medicare Medical Review—Home Health  P.O. Box 2019
Milwaukee, WI 53201-2019

Medicare Medical Review

1515 NORTH RIVER CENTER DRIVE ▼ P.O. BOX 2019 ▼ MILWAUKEE, WI 53201-2019 ▼ 414/226-5000
FEDERAL MEDICARE INTERMEDIARY

**FIGURE 5.4**

definitions is one of the contributing factors that permit the government and payers to broadly, and chaotically, interpret standards and conditions.

## Outcomes and Satisfaction

Quantitative data analysis of the benefits of home care is rudimentary and rather unsophisticated when it comes to patient outcomes and satisfaction. The industry as a whole has no foundation on which to base its claims of improved patient outcomes and satisfaction as a result of home care intervention. In order to truly make a case for the cost benefit of home care, at a minimum the two parameters of outcomes and satisfaction must be analyzed by

- primary diagnosis
- surgical procedure
- secondary diagnosis
- age
- sex
- living arrangements
- number of unexpected rehospitalizations for the primary diagnosis within a finite period after admission to home care

For smaller agencies this type of data can be gathered using conventional manual systems. For larger agencies the only reliable method of capturing this data is through a truly integrated data base capable of this type analysis. At the end of 1994, there was no commercially available, fully integrated, automated system for outcome measurements. Stand-alones developed by individual agencies were just emerging, as well as a few commercially available software products, but nothing answered the need for true outcome measurement analysis.

The need to accurately and objectively measure the outcomes of patients receiving home care will become more acute in the immediate future. As agencies apply pressure on software vendors for outcome data, the industry should expect an explosion of automated outcome measurement products.

# ONE METHOD TO DEVELOP OUTCOME MEASUREMENTS

While waiting for automated, integrated, outcome measurement data systems to become a reality, the home care industry cannot stand still. Having worked in and observed the health care service system during the past twenty-eight years, the author has concluded that for reasons unknown, there is a tendency within the health care service system to make relatively simple things complex, *and* require that the first attempt be perfect. Such is the reality of outcome measurements. What is offered in this section is a simple system with which to get started. Modification and refinements can be made *after* the system has been used for a few months. Figure 5.5 is a sample outcome measurement tool adapted from information presented at *Vision 2000 Home Care* in Boston on August 23, 1994.

# THE TOOL

This section is divided into four parts: *admission status/projected, projected visits/weeks, goal attainment date,* and *discharge status/projected.* The patient and significant other (S/O) are evaluated in each section that applies.

## Admission Status/Projected

At the time of admission, the nurse or therapist evaluates the patient in the goal categories of

- health status
- knowledge
- skills (short- and/or long-term)
- psychosocial
- if appropriate, the S/O's knowledge and skill

A score from 1 to 5 is given for each item assessed in the category. If both the patient and S/O are evaluated in the category of *knowledge,* the score for the patient would be recorded in the appropriate column with an *A* and the S/O with a *B.* If both the patient and S/O have the same score, it would be recorded as A/B in the appropriate column. Figure 5.6 is a sample of a completed tool, and can be referred to for visualization of the scoring procedure.

One-word scoring definitions are found at the bottom of the tool. At the time of admission, if a patient was evaluated at a score of 2 (suboptimal) in cognitive ability, found under *health status goals,* and the therapist expected the patient to reach 4 (functional) by discharge, it would be recorded as 2/4. To the left of each item assessed is a HCFA code for 485 and physician order production; to the right of each item is space where the therapist can record a brief patient-specific note relating to the item assessed.

## Projected Visits/Weeks

The plan is written out as *X* weeks over *Y* visits. If the nurse or therapist estimates the patient and S/O will be able to accomplish a particular skill in four weeks and eight visits, it would be written as 4/8 next to the corresponding item.

## Goal Attainment Date

When the patient reaches the projected goal, the date is entered. If the patient does not attain the goal(s), *not met* would be entered and an explanation made in the clinical progress note and/or case coordinator's narrative. Obviously, goals may change during

# FUNCTIONAL STATUS ASSESSMENT and GOALS FOR PHYSICAL THERAPY

Patient Name: _____  Patient ID# _____  SOC Date _____

Initial Assessment Date _____  Physical Therapy Discharge Date _____

| Goals for Home Care Physical Therapy | Functional Status Assessment | | | | |
|---|---|---|---|---|---|
| **B500** | Admission Status/ Projected | Projected visits/ weeks | Goal Attain Date | Dischg status/ projected | |
| **I. HEALTH STATUS GOALS**<br>IMPROVEMENT IN:<br>B501—Cognitive ability _____<br>B502—Activity/Energy level _____<br>B503—Tolerance to treatment _____<br>B504—Pain level _____<br>B505—Endurance _____<br>B506—OTHER _____ | | | | | |
| **2. KNOWLEDGE GOALS**<br>COMPETENCE OF CAREGIVER/PATIENT IN:<br>B521—Home safety _____<br>B522—ADL _____<br>B523—Transfers and Ambulation _____<br>B524—Home Exercise Program/Stump Care _____<br>B525—Equipment _____<br>B526—OTHER _____ | | | | | |
| **3. SKILLS GOALS—SHORT TERM**<br>B541—Bed/wheelchair mobility _____<br>B542—Transfers to tub/commode/toilet/shower/bed/chair with-without assistance _____<br>B543—Improve gross coordination of (extremity) _____<br>B544—Increase active/passive range of motion (degrees) _____<br>B545—Increase muscle strength (grade) _____<br>B546—Ambulation on level/uneven surface (ft assist.) _____<br>B547—Stair negotiation (steps/flights) _____<br>B548—OTHER _____ | | | | | |

## 4. SKILL GOALS—LONG TERM

B561—Bed/wheelchair mobility _____

B562—Transfers to tub/commode/toilet/shower/ bed chair with-without assistance _____

B563—Improve gross coordination of (extremity) _____

B564—Increase active/passive range of motion (degrees) _____

B565—Increase muscle strength (grade) _____

B566—Ambulation on level/uneven surface (steps/flight) _____

B567—Stair negotiation (steps/flight) _____

B568—OTHER _____

## 5. PSYCHOSOCIAL GOALS

IMPROVEMENT IN:

B581—Mental Status _____

B582—Motivation _____

B583—Self-concept _____

B584—Social isolation _____

B585—Confidence _____

B586—OTHER _____

## FUNCTIONAL STATUS CATEGORIES:

| | 1 | 2 | 3 | 4 | 5 |
|---|---|---|---|---|---|
| Health Status | Declining | Sub-optimal | Improving | Functional | Independent |
| Knowledge | Absent | Negligible | Adequate | Substantial | Competent |
| Skills | No Skill | Minimal Skill | Moderate Skill | Substantial Skill | Independent |
| Psychosocial | Decompensating | Sub-optimal | Improving | Functional | Resolved |

I:\USERS\SHAREALL\FUNCTPT.WPD

**FIGURE 5.5** (Reprinted with permission of Montefiore Medical Center Home Health Agency.)

# FUNCTIONAL STATUS ASSESSMENT and GOALS FOR PHYSICAL THERAPY

**Patient Name:** JOHN DOE  **Patient ID#** 916652  **SOC Date:** 020194

**Initial Assessment Date** 020194  **Physical Therapy Discharge Date** 022594

| Goals for Home Care Physical Therapy<br><br>B500 | Functional Status Assessment | | | |
|---|---|---|---|---|
| | Admission Status/ Projected | Projected visits/ weeks | Goal Attain Date | Dischg status/ projected |
| **1. HEALTH STATUS GOALS**<br>IMPROVEMENT IN:<br>B501—Cognitive ability<br>B502—Activity/Energy level<br>B503—Tolerance to treatment<br>B504—Pain level<br>B505—Endurance<br>B506—OTHER | 2/4 | 9/4 | 0218 | 4/4 |
| **2. KNOWLEDGE GOALS**<br>COMPETENCE OF CAREGIVER/PATIENT IN:<br>B521—Home safety<br>B522—ADL<br>B523—Transfers and Ambulation<br>B524—Home Exercise Program/Stump Care<br>B525—Equipment<br>B526—OTHER | 2/4 | 8/3 | 0218 | 4/4 |
| **3. SKILL GOALS—SHORT TERM**<br>B541—Bed/wheelchair mobility<br>B542—Transfers to tub/commode/toilet/shower/bed/chair with without assistance<br>B543—Improve gross coordination of (extremity)<br>B544—Increase active/passive range of motion (degrees) within functional limits<br>B545—Increase muscle strength (grade)<br>B546—Ambulation on level/uneven surface (ft assist.) 100 feet<br>B547—Stair negotiation (steps/flights)<br>B548—OTHER | 2/4<br>2/4<br><br>2/4 | 2/1<br>4/2<br><br>2/1 | 0204<br>0209<br><br>0207 | 4/4<br>4/4<br><br>4/4 |

MAJOR JOINT REPLACE-
MENT RT HIP

## 4. SKILL GOALS—LONG TERM

| | | | | |
|---|---|---|---|---|
| B561—Bed/wheelchair mobility | | | | |
| B562—Transfers to tub/commode/toilet/shower/ bed chair with~without~ assistance | 2/5 | 11/4 | 0221 | 5/5 |
| B563—Improve gross coordination of (extremity) | | | | |
| B564—Increase active/passive range of motion (degrees) | | | | |
| B565—Increase muscle strength (grade) | | | | |
| B566—Ambulation on level/uneven surface (steps/flight) 100 feet | 1/5 | 11/4 | 0228 | 4/5 |
| B567—Stair negotiation (steps/flight) | | | | |
| B568—OTHER | | | | |

## 5. PSYCHOSOCIAL GOALS

IMPROVEMENT IN:

| | | | | |
|---|---|---|---|---|
| B581—Mental Status | | | | |
| B582—Motivation | | | | |
| B583—Self-concept | | | | |
| B584—Social isolation | | | | |
| B585—Confidence in ability to independently ambulate | 2/5 | 11/4 | 0228 | 4/5 |
| B586—OTHER | | | | |

**FUNCTIONAL STATUS CATEGORIES:**

| | 1 | 2 | 3 | 4 | 5 |
|---|---|---|---|---|---|
| Health Status | Declining | Sub-optimal | Improving | Functional | Independent |
| Knowledge | Absent | Negligible | Adequate | Substantial | Competent |
| Skills | No Skill | Minimal Skill | Moderate Skill | Substantial Skill | Independent |
| Psychosocial | Decompensating | Sub-optimal | Improving | Functional | Resolved |

**FIGURE 5.6** (Reprinted with permission of Montefiore Medical Center Home Health Agency.)

the course of treatment. Modifications should be reflected on the tool and in the clinical progress notes.

## Discharge Status/Projected

At the time of discharge, the patient and S/O are evaluated in the same categories they were evaluated in at admission and the score is recorded. The discharge score is recorded *over* the projected. For instance, if the patient scores 3 in health status but a score of 4 had been projected, it would be recorded as 3/4.

## Difference

The difference between discharge status and projected indicates how successful the patient was in attaining the goals set out at the time of initial assessment. A numeric and subsequent percentage value can be determined to demonstrate improvement. For example, if a patient demonstrated poor self-esteem (score 1) at admission as a result of disfiguring surgery, and at the time of discharge scored 3, there would have been a 200 percent improvement in self-esteem.

Again refer to Figure 5.6, which illustrates an outcome tool for a patient with a major joint replacement.

## Tracking Outcomes and Utilization

The quality management department should be the main group responsible for investigation and compilation of outcome data and subsequent utilization review analysis. Once sufficient data has been garnered, it must be shared with

- clinical management and staff
- financial managers
- intake staff
- senior management

With reliable and validated outcome projections, the agency can use the findings to quantify to any number of entities the physical, emotional, and social progress and improvement made by patients and families. Obviously, this is an ongoing process that requires permanent assignment of resources and personnel to track and evaluate the organization's successes in maintaining or improving patient outcomes.

# BENEFITS OF OUTCOME MEASURES

The benefits of outcome measures are many, and are listed below.

- Objective analysis of the care rendered can be made via a quantitative value index.
- The amount of time in weeks and the number of visits necessary to accomplish the goals developed at the time of admission are clear.

- As the data base is developed, the average number of weeks and visits necessary to care for a particular diagnosis can be established.
- Once average length of stay and visit consumption have been confirmed, agency staffing patterns can be more accurately developed and budgeted.
- Meeting the present, and future, requirements of regulatory and accreditation bodies for reporting objective patient outcomes.
- The development of critical pathways for the most common home care diagnoses is obtainable.
- Reliable statistical data from which to negotiate managed care contracts or capitation agreements are available.

Outcome measurement lends itself well to some form of an automated data system that can be sorted and evaluated on a number of parameters. The commercial market does not have a wealth of providers producing such products. For obvious reasons it would be best if the industry were to develop it, rather than the payers, regulators, or surveyors.

# CONCLUSION

TQM and CQI both lead to outcome measurements. An entire patient-focused TQM and CQI program can be built around such measurements. Also, the concept of outcome measures can be adapted to the operational (nonclinical) aspects of the agency through nonclinical CQI committees.

The importance of simplicity and ease of use cannot be stressed enough. As the application of outcome measures becomes more familiar, it will *naturally* evolve to encompass more sophisticated tools to predict and measure the quality of care delivered or operational efficiency of the organization.

Outcome measures for home care are in the formative phase. Trying to make the process perfect on the first or second attempt is not a realistic objective. Because the process is in such an early stage, there is little resource material available to guide an agency in the development of outcome measurement.

Forces outside the industry are compelling rapid development of outcome measures. If the industry does not develop them, someone or something else will. A word of caution—rushing into poorly designed outcomes has the potential to be more disastrous than not having any at all.

## *Suggested Readings*

Davis, E. R. (1994). *Total quality management for home care.* Gathersburg, MD: Aspen Publishers, Inc.

Koch, M. W., & Fairly, T. M. (1993). *Integrated quality management the key to improving nursing care quality.* St. Louis, MO: Mosby.

Joint Commission on Accreditation of Healthcare Organizations. (1994). *1995 accreditation manual for home health care.* Oakbrook, IL: JCAHO.

Joint Commission on Accreditation of Healthcare Organizations. (1992). *Using quality improvement tools in a healthcare setting.* Oakbrook, IL: JCAHO.

Joint Commission on Accreditation of Healthcare Organizations. (1993). *Quality improvement in home care.* Oakbrook, IL: JCAHO.

Wilson, A. (1993, June). Bridging cost & quality through patient outcome measurement. *CARING Magazine,* pp. 40–44.

Wilson, A. (1993). Managed Competition. *Nursing Administration Quarterly,* 17(4), 11–16.

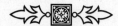

# CHAPTER

# Selected Legal Issues in Home Health Care

**Robert W. Gunther**

In the United States, home health care agencies (HHAs) face a wide variety of legal liabilities in the 1990s. Significant change in health care law is only a possibility. The Clinton Administration has begun a legislative process to produce a national health reform program by the fall of 1995. This may have an effect on HHA practices with regard to their potential liability, but the final result, if any, is not known.

Presently, however, liability exposure for HHAs include civil malpractice and negligence claims by HHA patients, and administrative and even criminal actions by state and federal governmental entities. The reference list for this chapter, although not encyclopedic, provides several resources that cover these and numerous other subjects more thoroughly.

# CIVIL LIABILITY

Although most malpractice claims have arisen in the hospital or physician's office setting, home health care providers are also being held responsible for malpractice. There may be several causes for civil litigation against HHAs. One is that the role of the HHA has grown.

Today the HHA provider's function includes delivery of highly technological services to patients who may have been discharged from hospitals "sicker and quicker," and therefore have an increased chance of poor outcomes. Second, home health care services are provided in individuals' homes, where the environment is somewhat uncontrollable. Direct supervision is less available in the home than in a hospital or nursing home setting; patient compliance is harder to achieve. These and other factors have resulted in increasing liability exposure for HHAs.

In several states, legal exposure for malpractice in home health care has broadened to include corporate liability. Corporate liability can be found where there is a nondelegable duty owed by the HHA to the patient that requires the HHA to exercise reasonable care to ensure that a patient receives competent care. The HHA's duties in this respect require that it comply with the standard of a competent HHA acting in the same or similar circumstances.

Corporate liability is triggered when malpractice occurs that could have been prevented by the proper screening, evaluating, or training of staff members. In applying the standard of care, courts may consider state licensing and certification laws, the HHA's own procedures, and Joint Commission on Accreditation of Healthcare Organizations (JCAHO) or Community Healthcare Accreditation Program (CHAP) standards.

### Case Study

An illustrative example of a home health care malpractice action that involved corporate liability is the case of *Dickman v. City of New York* (1991). An 80-year-old woman suffered a fractured hip when she fell in her home while being attended by a New York City home health care worker. The plaintiff was hospitalized for three months and was permanently bedridden. She alleged that the HHA failed to properly train, hire, and supervise its personnel. The claim was settled for $350,000. Incidentally, the predicted range of a jury verdict in favor of the plaintiff in the New York City Borough of Queens, where the action was brought, was $200,000 to $500,000.

A case from Oregon, *Roach v. Kelly Health Care* (1987), is a principal case involving home care malpractice in the United States. Here, the court held that determining the standard of care applying to a certified agency required consideration of Oregon's home health care regulations. In this case the agency had been required by Oregon health laws to provide its patients with home health aides as opposed to certified nursing assistants (CNAs), but failed to do so. Instead, the HHA had provided CNAs.

This was significant to the court because the aides would have received more training than the CNAs and been expected to confer at the home office to review the patient's treatment. The failure to do so was found to be negligence by law. Therefore the court instructed the jury that it could conclude that the CNAs were not qualified to provide the health care services required by statute, making it easier for the plaintiff to prove her case against the HHA.

The court also found that the HHA had improperly delegated administrative and supervisory functions to the Visiting Nurse Association (VNA), which was also providing home care to the patient and had not established proper written procedures to prevent the occurrence. The jury found that the actions of the defendant HHA and VNA contributed to the injuries of the patient. The jury also found that the CNAs were confused as to whether they were to report to their supervisors or to the VNA nurses, and that the HHA supervisors were responsible for instructing the HHA CNAs at the time.

*Roach* indicates that when determining if there may be HHA malpractice, a court may consider applicable regulations prescribing structural aspects of quality control, which tend to be within the expertise of the HHA, as evidence of the applicable standard of care. Standards falling within this category include the implementation of procedures and policies concerning training and placement of care givers, maintenance of records, and monitoring of care given and incidents arising during the course of that care.

# VICARIOUS LIABILITY

An HHA may be held vicariously liable for the malpractice of its staff for treatment of home care patients below the standard of care. A patient harmed through the malpractice of an HHA may recover against it by proving that the HHA employee caused the injury and was acting within the scope of employment.

*Tomlinson, Estate of v. Underhill Personnel Services* (1988) is a Florida case that applied the law of vicarious liability. A 59-year-old attorney suffered a femur fracture while under the care of the defendant HHA's employee. The plaintiff alleged that the defendant's employee knew he was not able to stand alone, and her negligence caused his injury. The plaintiff retained as an expert witness a radiation oncologist, while the defense retained a nursing expert. The plaintiff received $125,000 for pain and suffering and $9,600 for medical expenses.

In *Freeman, Estate of v. Upjohn Health Care: Derr; Hess* (1990), an 18-month-old infant died after being under the care of defendant HHA nurses. The infant had numerous medical problems and was respirator dependent. The plaintiff alleged that the HHA nurses failed to properly monitor the infant and thereby allowed the respirator to clog with mucus, which caused the infant's death. The defendant HHA asserted in its defense that the infant's rare muscular disease instead had caused end stage lung disease, resulting in her death. The plaintiff had retained a nursing expert witness while the defense had a pathologist prepared to testify on its behalf. The adverse jury award potential was $50,000 to $100,000. The claim settled before trial for $50,000.

**Case Study**

In *Jones v. Upjohn Health Care Services* (1991), the defendant HHA received a defense verdict. An 85-year-old male suffered third-degree burns to his foot, allegedly during a bath that he received from an employee of the defendant HHA. The plaintiff required skin grafting and the decedent's wife alleged he died one month later because of the burns.

The case was tried only on the issue of vicarious liability of the HHA for the employee's malpractice. The plaintiff alleged the employee was negligent for retaining an employee who it knew, or should have known, was reprimanded and terminated by another employer for patient abuse.

The defendant HHA asserted that the bath was not witnessed by anyone and that the patient's complaints of burns were initiated by his wife. The plaintiff responded that the decedent had immediately reported that his foot had been burned following the bath.

The HHA's expert medical witness, who was a vascular surgeon, testified that the decedent's wounds were not caused by burns but instead by his underlying vascular and arterial disease. The plaintiff had no expert witnesses to testify in support of its claim. The plaintiff's final pre-trial demand was $180,000 while the HHA only offered $30,000.

Courts may liberally interpret the scope of an employee's conduct, which may even be deemed to include unauthorized or even specifically disapproved actions. Generally speaking, the HHA staff is not negligent when they follow physicians' treatment orders unless they are aware that the orders are incorrect or a present danger to the patient.

# INDEPENDENT CONTRACTORS

An HHA may even be found vicariously liable for the malpractice of independent contractors who cause injury to the patient. This is because courts are expected to increasingly identify that it is the duty of the HHA to monitor the competency of its independent contractors. This duty may be found, for example, in private or governmental accreditation standards.

Generally, an independent contractor performs specific care services and controls the manner in which these services are provided. Normally, the independent contractor may control when the service is to be provided, is responsible for travel and business expenses, and may receive a 1099 IRS form instead of a W-2 for documentation of his or her compensation.

Additionally, courts may apply the theory of apparent, or ostensible, agency to hold HHAs liable for the malpractice of independent contractors. Under apparent agency theory, the independent contractor is held to be an agent of the HHA because he or she reasonably appears to be acting under the authority of the HHA.

With this potential liability exposure in mind, an HHA should seek to minimize liability exposure by closely monitoring its marketing publications for any express or implied representations with regard to its relationship with independent contractors. "The vicarious liability provided by ostensible agency provides a much broader basis for liability than does an independent duty to monitor the quality of direct caregivers, or other similar structural duties." (Johnson, 1991).

# ABANDONMENT

Liability will be imposed upon an HHA for the negligent discharge or transfer of a patient to another treatment facility. Normally, an HHA should consider the propriety of a transfer or discharge before doing so. However, with the possibility that some form of a prospective payment system will be instituted for home health care, negligent referral, transfer, or discharge may become a larger temptation. A home care transfer should never put the patient at risk.

A number of legal cases have been reported in which a transfer, resulting in exacerbation of a patient's condition, was found to be an abandonment. Under the law, abandonment can be found when there is a unilateral termination of the HHA's relationship with the patient without reasonable motive or proper notice when the patient's condition necessitates continuing attention.

A claim of abandonment is based on the breach of the contractual relationship that the HHA has with the patient. Once the HHA agrees to treat the patient, the HHA should continue to provide services until

- the services are no longer reasonably required
- the HHA is discharged by the patient
- there is mutual agreement to terminate the relationship
- the HHA has been replaced by another competent HHA
- the HHA has been otherwise relieved

In the physician's office setting, for example, the analysis of whether a continuing patient physician relationship exists is easier to determine. There is usually a mutual agreement that the doctor is committed to treating the patient through the course of the illness or until services are no longer needed. There are a large number of court decisions reported in every state that enforce the agreement to provide continuing care.

Before a physician may withdraw from a patient's care there are two requirements that must be satisfied by the physician. First, the patient or family must receive adequate notice that care will be discontinued. And second, the patient or family must be given ample opportunity to find substitute care. It is likely that HHAs will similarly be required to provide their patients with notice and time to secure alternative services.

Courts may apply the doctrine of abandonment to HHAs when a patient becomes noncompliant, the home setting becomes unsafe, or reimbursement is denied (Johnson, 1991). Liability for abandoning a patient may also apply to HHAs when home care services are withheld because of suspected lack of reimbursement. In addition, states are addressing the issues of unsafe conditions, especially in the inner city, and the HHA's responsibility to provide care in situations where the staff's safety and welfare are potentially jeopardized (NYCRR-10, 1994).

**Case Study**

In *Ready v. Personal Health Care Services; Community Psychiatric Centers* (1991), a 3-year-old boy was under the care of the defendant HHA. The care was unilaterally terminated by the HHA on the alleged grounds that the plaintiff's insurer refused to continue payment because it was no longer medically necessary. The boy died of pneumonia within three months of home care service termination.

The boy's father and mother instituted legal action for severe emotional distress, which they allegedly developed because of their son's death. The father contended that his insurance company had not refused payment, but that the HHA had incorrectly determined that the plaintiff was only insured for $50,000, so the HHA terminated home care services when the boy's home care bill reached $49,425. At trial, the plaintiff presented expert testimony from a psychiatrist, social worker, and pediatric nurse. The psychiatrist's testimony was given to support the plaintiffs' alleged injuries of emotional distress, while the nurse testified as to the deviation from the standard of acceptable care that the HHA committed.

The defendant HHA contended that the insurer had refused payment and that the boy could have died even with continued home health care. The defendant HHA presented testimony from a pediatrician, pulmonologist, pediatric neurologist, and nurse. The physicians' testimony was presented by the HHA to give their opinions that the infant's underlying condition caused his death, not the HHA's withdrawal of its services. The HHA's nurse expert testified that the standard of care as it applied to the HHA's withdrawal of treatment was arguably acceptable.

The plaintiff's pre-trial demand was $350,000, while the HHA's insurer made no counteroffer. The jury awarded the mother $1,500,000 for compensatory damages, $405,000 for special damages, and $5,850,000 for punitive damages. The jury awarded the father $500,000 for compensatory damages, $381,000 for special damages, and also $5,850,000 for punitive damages. Punitive damages are not normally insurable because the courts have held that it would be against public policy to provide indemnity for negligence or malpractice that warrants punishment. Otherwise, the jury's verdict of imposing punitive damages would be subject to being undercut.

Documentation of discharge planning by the HHA is an important risk management policy consideration. An HHA should consider using a discharge planning form that patients must sign, and document behavioral progress notes in the patients' records concerning their ability to engage in certain behaviors on their own prior to discharge (Hartz & Bucalo, 1987).

# PATIENT'S RIGHT TO REFUSE TREATMENT

A home care patient's refusal of treatment can be a form of unilateral discharge. Under the doctrine of informed consent, treatment may not be performed on a patient without that patient's consent. An HHA is required to adequately inform the patient of the nature of the proposed treatment. This must include a discussion of the risks, benefits, and alternatives.

However, the right of a competent person to refuse treatment is not absolute. Most states also have the right under the law to preserve life, protect third parties, and prevent suicide. This presents a conflict, a need to balance the interests between the state's and the individual's rights. An example of this is presently unfolding in Michigan, where Dr. Jack Kervorkian is repeatedly assisting terminally ill individuals in committing suicide despite a recently enacted Michigan law that which forbids assisted suicide.

Determining the patient's competency to refuse treatment may sometimes be quite difficult. If there is any question as to the patient's competency to refuse treatment, a professional consultation must be performed and a documented opinion obtained. Some patients may not refuse all treatments, but only selected treatments or procedures. Selective refusals of treatment may complicate the patient's care (Johnson, 1991).

An incompetent patient's right to refuse medical care requires the court to determine who may make the decision and on what basis. Many courts have used the "substituted standard," which requires the decision maker to decide as the patient would be expected to. For this the decision maker must take into consideration the patient's ethics and experiences that would reveal what the patient's decision would be.

Other courts may use the "best interests" standard to decide whether to refuse treatments. Here the decision maker would consider the benefits versus the burden of the treatment.

In reality, medical and legal procedures are significantly different. Health care staff reportedly consult and rely on a patient's spouse or adult offspring. If the patient has no living will or health care proxy, most state laws require a legally appointed guardian. After a legal guardian has been appointed, it must be decided under what circumstances a decision may be made to refuse medical treatment without a court's involvement (Johnson, 1991).

A 1986 New Jersey case considered this issue (*In the Matter of Kathleen Farrell*, 1987). A 37-year-old, respirator-dependent, home care patient requested to be disconnected. The patient's husband sought to be appointed guardian and a court hearing and psychological examination of the patient were conducted. A year after the patient's death, the New Jersey Supreme Court issued its opinion, on behalf of future cases. The court balanced the individual's rights versus the state's interests and found the patient's interests superior.

The *Farrell* court also proposed procedures for refusal of treatment by competent home care patients in the future. First, the patient must be found to be competent and properly informed about his or her prognosis, the alternative treatments available, and the risk involved in the withdrawal of the life-sustaining treatment. Second, the patient's decision must be completely voluntary and uncoerced. Two nonattending physicians must be of the opinion that the patient is competent and fully informed of all relevant matters. Last, the patient's rights must be balanced against the state's interests.

Some legal authorities on HHAs believe that "the court would have better served the patients and healthcare professionals had it simply held that the state's interests, perhaps except in the case of a parent of young children, do not outweigh the right of a competent patient to refuse medical treatment" (Johnson, 1991).

However, the court indicated that it should not be necessary for a court to routinely intervene in the case of refusal of treatment by competent home care patients. The court decided that it would become involved to resolve disputes in and among the physician(s), family and/or other health care providers.

The court also indicated that no person would incur civil or criminal liability who, in good faith reliance on the procedures established in the opinion, withdraws life-sustaining treatment at the request of an informed and competent patient, if the patient has an independent medical examination.

Besides fearing the possibility of liability exposure for complying with a patient's refusal of treatment, health care providers also risk liability for *failing* to comply with a patient's request. Patients and their families have brought claims against health care facilities for continuing treatment despite the patient's, or representative's, refusal of consent for the treatment.

## High Tech Issues

Highly sophisticated, technologically advanced equipment is increasingly being utilized to treat home care patients. In addition to the manufacturers, vendors, and suppliers of the equipment, HHAs face liability exposure for injuries caused by any defect or misuse of the equipment.

Primary service providers of sophisticated medical equipment in the home may be the suppliers, while the HHA staff performs a secondary role. As noted in the *Roach v. Kelly Health Care* (1987) case, coordination of treatment plans and clear lines of authority are required to prevent the HHA from being potentially liable for the injuries caused by medical equipment.

Plaintiffs may use various theories of liability, including negligent prescription, design, manufacture, installation, maintenance, or repair of medical equipment. Plaintiffs normally use several theories in a claim for injuries caused by medical equipment and include as many different parties as possible.

## Case Study

In *Long v. Sci-O-Tech, Inc.* (1992), a quadriplegic suffered emotional distress and posttraumatic stress disorder when the head broke on the electrical bed he purchased from the codefendant home health care (home medical equipment) vendor, manufactured by the defendant company. The head of the bed fell from an inclined position, approximately 1 1/2 feet. The plaintiff contended that the defendant was negligent for manufacturing a defective product, and that the codefendant home health care (home medical equipment) vendor was negligent for selling a defective product.

The defendants denied that the bed was defective, and contended that the codefendant was negligent for making changes to the bed. The vendor denied any negligence and both defendants denied that the plaintiff suffered any injuries. Only the home health care (home medical equipment) vendor was liable for the $10,000 verdict.

## Case Study

In *Higley v. Crow River Industries; Home Health, Inc.* (1991), a 3-year-old suffered a head injury resulting in facial and arm paralysis and speech dysfunction after his head became caught within a moving mechanism of a wheelchair lift on the defendant transportation service's van.

The plaintiff claimed that the defendant transportation service was negligent in allowing small children to ride close to dangerous machinery without adequate safeguards, not providing proper training of its employees in the use of the equipment, and not providing training in emergency procedures. The plaintiff claimed that Home Health Inc., which installed and serviced the lift, was strictly liable for the product it sold because it failed to distribute the instruction manual and necessary tools for safe lift operation.

The boy's mother and sisters, who witnessed the accident, claimed to have suffered emotional distress. The plaintiff also named the manufacturer of the lift as a defendant, claiming it was improperly manufactured. A structured settlement was agreed upon for payments over thirty years with an anticipated payout of $4,858,759.

An HHA may also face vicarious liability for the injuries caused by medical equipment, based on not only the vendor's duty to perform customary or required services, but also based on any services the vendor undertakes on its own.

In *Ardoin v. Hartford Accident and Indemnity* (1977), the plaintiff's estate sued a manufacturer who sold a hospital a heart-lung machine, as well as sued the hospital itself. During open heart surgery, the hospital perfusionist received incorrect information from the vendor, which caused the patient's death. The jury found the perfusionist and vendor negligent and held the hospital vicariously liable for negligence.

# GOVERNMENTAL LIABILITY

HHAs are subject to state regulation through required licensure and federal regulations if the HHA participates in Medicare (M/C) or Medicaid (M/A) programs. Participation in M/C is voluntary, but licensure of HHAs is normally mandatory.

Governmental enforcement of home health care rules and regulations can involve any of the following.

- revocation of the HHA's license
- suspension of admissions
- public monitoring
- receivership
- injunction
- fines
- criminal penalties
- no action (Johnson, 1989)

Home health agencies are also liable to investigations by the U.S. Department of Justice, state insurance commissioners, and law enforcement agencies, besides state licensing boards. A state may follow the federal government's enforcement practices or its own, even if the standards to be applied are identical.

State licensing statutes vary. Several state statutes regulating HHAs are based on the federal government's statutes governing M/C. The relevant M/C statute 42 U.S.C. §1395x (o)(i), enacted in 1982, provides that M/C regulations require that a certified home health agency (CHHA) provide "[p]art-time or intermittent skilled nursing services and at least one other therapeutic service."

Some states have enacted legislation governing HHAs that does not follow the federal statutes. For example, the District of Columbia defines an HHA for purposes of licensure as: an agency, organization or distinct part thereof, other than a hospital that provides either directly or through a contractual arrangement, a program of health care, habilitative or rehabilitative therapy, personal care services, homemaker services, chore services or other supportive services to sick or disabled individuals living at home or in a community residence facility. (D.C. Code Ann §32-1301(a), 1986)

## Imposition of Fines

At least five states and the District of Columbia have authority to levy civil fines against HHAs: Minnesota, Montana, Pennsylvania, Texas, and Illinois. Fines have the effect of increasing the cost of operating the HHA and decreasing the benefit of providing or attempting to provide substandard home health care.

Fines can be imposed that address the severity of the violation and the underlying economic incentives. Fines are especially appropriate for violations that involve only a few patients, if the violation is not expected to be repeated. Prior to judicial court proceedings, most states provide for administrative agency procedures and hearings. Administrative proceedings generally may be less severe than formal court hearings, which could involve extensive delays, including appeals.

Administrative procedures have the flexibility of providing an informal conference setting to resolve the imposition of a civil fine or a full administrative hearing. If a formal administrative hearing is held, a complete transcript of the proceedings should be requested in the event an HHA later needs to seek legal protection. Legal protection would prevent the court, at the time of a subsequent trial, from considering any remedial improvements by the HHA following the occurrence that originally gave rise to the administrative attention or action. In other words, positive steps taken by the HHA to correct the deficiency(s) that led to the action could not be used to "prove" the guilt of the agency.

The purpose of the threat or imposition of civil fines is to seek to obtain compliance by the HHA with the state's rules and regulations. More important than the monetary loss that an administrative fine may represent is the effect that any publicity would have on the reputation of the agency.

## Suspension of Service

Another enforcement action that the state may take against an HHA is the suspension of the agency's patient care services. Suspending patient admissions could apply to both M/C certified and private pay agencies. Normally, if a state imposes a suspension of admissions to an HHA, the state should notify the current patients and their attending physicians.

This notice should include a telephone hot line to call for additional information. For those HHA patients who desire to transfer to another agency, the state should provide some form of discharge planning. The state's responsibility to provide this action is to prevent a patient from being placed in the compromising position of seeking to change agencies, yet not wanting to offend the agency on which the action is being taken.

## Receivership

A state may also place an HHA in receivership. A state agency most likely would seek implementation of this provision when the HHA appeared likely to close without providing continued care for its patients. Additionally, the regulating agency may seek this administrative sanction when there is a serious violation and little evidence that the HHA is seeking to correct the situation.

This administrative remedy would be most suitable in rural settings where no other HHA services are available. More importantly, the state should require the HHA to provide notice to its patients and their physicians, oversee the transfer of records, and provide information regarding acceptable alternatives.

## Fraud and Abuse

Home health agencies are susceptible to being excluded from M/C and M/A certification if they are found to have committed fraud. The U.S. Department of Health and Human Services (DHHS) Office of the Inspector General (OIG) has brought twenty-three fraud and abuse proceedings against HHAs under the M/C and M/A programs, and excluded sixteen HHAs from the M/C program (Commercial Appeal, 1992).

The OIG is increasing utilization of criminal statutes to prosecute health care fraud and abuse. These federal laws include, but are not limited to the following.

- conspiracy to defraud the United States
- false statements
- false, fictitious, or fraudulent claims
- theft or bribery
- impeding a federal auditor
- failure to disclose ownership/control information (Pyles, 1993)

There are several strategic advantages for the federal government to utilize criminal statutes vis-à-vis M/C enforcement statutes. One of these advantages permits the U.S. Department of Justice to prosecute HHAs for criminal violations, which are easier to prove than federal M/C violations.

Previously, inadequacies in the OIG's survey and inspection process may have been caused by inadequate budget allocations and responsibilities for inspection of providers other than HHAs. However, the Health Care Financing Administration (HFCA) has significantly increased the OIG's budget for HHA survey in order to increase the number and frequency of surveys. According to the OIG's report of September, 1987, HHA decertification proceedings were the only sanctions available because surveyors had failed to cite HHAs for violations during the survey process. Because decertification was such a drastic measure, only a few decertification proceedings had been undertaken. In order to remedy this, the 1987 Budget Reconciliation Act authorized intermediate sanctions for HHAs under 42 USCA § 1395a.

## Survey and Inspection

Hand-in-hand with licensure of home health care agencies are surveys and inspections. A 1985 survey conducted by the National Association for Home Care (NAHC) revealed that 78 percent of the home health care providers reported M/C certification on-site inspections occurred annually. Seventy-five percent reported annual M/A on-site visits and 71 percent reported annual non-Medicare/Medicaid "visits." Most states conduct the M/C and licensure inspections at the same time (National Association for Home Care, 1985).

However, a 1985 report of the DHHS OIG also indicated that M/C certified home health agencies are not usually resurveyed annually. Among the sixteen home health agencies visited by the inspection team in 1986, only one had been surveyed in the previous year, five in 1985, seven in 1984, one in 1983, and two in 1981. The OIG further indicated in the same study that resurveys were backlogged one to four years and that branch offices of HHAs were not usually visited on resurvey (U.S. Department of Health & Human Services, 1987).

# CONCLUSION

Home health agencies operate with ever-increasing civil and governmental liability exposure. The major areas of risk and liability exposure have been reviewed. By no means has this review been exhaustive. The reader is advised, and would be well-rewarded, to continue to explore this area of law, as it has definite impact on the day-to-day practice, organization, and administration of home care.

# REFERENCES

*Ardoin v. Hartford Accident and Indemnity.* 1977. 350 So.2d 205 (La. App.).

*Commercial Appeal.* May 17, 1992. at B1, col. 1.

*Dickman v. City of New York.* 1991. WL 448689 (LRP).

*Freeman, Estate of v. Upjohn Health Care; Derr; Hess.* 1990. WL 466684, (LRP).

Hartz & Bucalo. (1987). Legal aspects of ethical issues in the continuum of care." *Managing the continuum of care.* Rockville, MD: Aspen Publishers.

*Higley v. Crow River Industries; Home Health, Inc.* 1991. WL 475523 (LRP).

*In the Matter of Kathleen Farrell.* 1987. 529 A.2d 404 (N.J.).

Johnson, S.H. (1991). Liability Issues. *Delivering high technology home care.* New York: Springer Publishing Co.

Johnson, S.H. (1989). Quality-control regulation of home health care. *Houston Law Review,* 26, 901.

*Jones v. Upjohn Health Care Services.* 1991. WL 447285, (LRP).

*Long v. Sci-O-Tech, Inc.; Glasrock Home Health Care,* 1992. WL 504725 (LRP).

National Association for Home Care. (1985). *Homecare quality assurance survey 9.*

New York Codes Rules and Regulations, 1994. (NYCRR-10) New York State Department of Health, Albany, N.Y., 1994.

Pyles, J.C. (1993). The increasing risk to home health providers under the antifraud and abuse laws. *Hospital home care strategic management for integrated care delivery.* Chicago: American Hospital Association.

*Ready v. Personal Health Care Services.* 1991. Community Psychiatric *Centers,* WL 448614 and 448615 (LRP).

*Roach v. Kelly Health Care.* 1987. 87 Or App. 495, 742 P. 2d. 1190.

*Tomlinson, Estate of v. Uderhill Personnel Services,* 1990 WL 457814, (LRP).

U.S. Department of Health & Human Services of the Inspector General. (1987). *Home health aide services for M/C patients.* Washington, D.C.: U.S. Government Printing Office.

# CHAPTER

# Empowering Employees for Excellence, Energy, and Enthusiasm

George D. Dugan
Susan Craig Schulmerich

The great dilemma we face in health care is this: we have a growing and aging patient population, too little money, and too much regulation. Once, everyone's parents were married forever, everybody's aunts and uncles lived near them and were visited frequently, almost every mother stayed home with the children, and nearly all elderly grandparents came to live and eventually die with the family. Today, parents are divorced, grandparents live in Florida, families are smaller and spread far apart, and few people can afford the luxury of a gradual slide into old age. Because more women work, elderly parents cannot simply be brought into the family residence; there is no one there to care for them. The number of elderly is growing impressively. Recent projections estimate that in the United States those over eighty-five will grow from 3.3 million today to between 18.7 and 72 million in 2080 (Kolata, 1992). At the same time, the whole country is concerned about our inability to pay for and control the cost of health care.

A large and growing demand for services, a belief in the patient's "right" to services, and the question of how to pay for those services create the dichotomy of health care. Home care managers will be challenged by an associated management dichotomy; handle a huge growth in patient demand with shrinking funds. Lessons from Japanese and American management leaders who have been developing new approaches to making their organizations efficient and productive are worth reviewing. Some of these approaches can be adapted to the health care industry and home care in particular. Each of these approaches has multiple ingredients which, when combined, make a complete process. The amalgamation of three approaches is the ultimate goal of the organization.

# NEW APPROACHES TO INCREASING EFFICIENCY AND PRODUCTIVITY

The first of these approaches is: *the organizational leader must personally create the vision of the highly productive agency and personally lead the effort to achieve it.* This may sound simple, but it is a profound point. The leadership of the *quality and productivity* effort cannot be delegated: it just will not work. According to The Japan Productivity Center, an important reason for the Japanese competitive success over the United States is that productivity is *the primary* job of the Japanese chief executive officer (CEO). In the U.S., however, quality is usually delegated to a vice president of productivity or some other senior executive.

The story of a recognized quality expert who was invited to speak to the senior management of one of America's largest companies being devastated by Japanese competition illustrates the importance of top management involvement. When the CEO rose and announced that a new senior executive would lead the productivity effort of the company, the invited expert got up and walked out. The "boss" failed to understand the single most important point: that he, himself, had to make quality his single most important objective and lead the company in a new way of operating. After a hasty private side meeting with the consultant, the CEO returned to the conference and announced he would personally lead the effort. Today that company is one of the most successful in the world.

There are three basic elements that must be instilled throughout the agency to achieve the new management approach of *organizational leadership personally creating the vision of the highly productive agency and leading the effort to achieve it.* Few organizations have been able to accomplish these three elements as a primary, unified goal. At best, they have focused on one or two. Even then, those that have followed through for the five or more years it takes to integrate them into an organization have had outstanding results.

## The Three Basic Elements

The first, *humanizing the work place,* empowers employees to contribute their best all day every day when management

1. treats employees with respect
2. builds mutual trust
3. opens two-way communication
4. improves job security
5. makes teamwork a habit
6. develops workers as problem solvers
7. moves toward worker self supervision
8. maintains a long-term consensus building approach toward managing the work force

The second, *improving patient care effectiveness,* delivers the best quality care at the lowest cost. This can be achieved by

1. developing a *culture* of continuous quality improvement in patient care
2. eliminating all waste in the delivery of care
3. reducing all thruput times to an absolute minimum
4. improving flexibility to respond to change

Last, *strategic patient service* can be realized by

1. making top-quality patient service a senior management priority
2. hiring and training super service oriented employees
3. improving complaint gathering and analysis methods
4. fixing all complaints quickly
5. fixing the system defect that caused the complaint
6. building a culture that leads employees to provide service "beyond their job"

# UNDERSTANDING EMPOWERMENT— MASLOW'S PYRAMID

The first factor in the triad, *humanizing the work place,* means continually empowering employees to contribute their best toward a directed team effort. Think back over your work life. Have you ever worked in a facility where you could fully utilize all of your skills and abilities? Do you as the manager provide a work environment where there are no barriers to employees doing their best? If the answer to either or both of these questions is "no," the work environment lacks empowerment and the resulting improved performance. Empowerment humanizes work, and when properly guided can contribute to continuously improved performance. Figure 7.1 is modeled after Maslow's hierarchy; each level in the pyramid will be reviewed.

## Respect

The best American organizations meet this challenge by establishing a climate of respect for each employee, and respect for the contribution that even the lowest paid employees can make to the organization. For example, at the transportation department of a large health care institution, the dispatcher had six patients waiting for wheelchairs and none were available. He suggested to his supervisor that they needed to buy some walkers to free up wheelchairs that were being hoarded on the units. The supervisor, instead of encouraging the idea, immediately said "we can't do that," giving reasons why he did not think it could be done.

Historically, there has been a lack of respect displayed by doctors toward nurses and by nurses toward nurse's aides or housekeepers, much as the child who has been punished turns and kicks the dog. We must treat each other respectfully every day. This can be achieved by both short- and long-term actions that include but are not limited to

- listening to others' problems and suggestions
- sharing information about the organization and its goals (especially information formerly treated as confidential) through multimedia communication
- eliminating the marks of special privilege that set people apart

## Trust

Trust, the second level of the pyramid, is at the heart of the Japanese management system. One method for management to build trust is by diligently and consistently fulfilling commitments to employees. Supervisors' actions can no longer be blindly supported. The "management right or wrong" philosophy has gone the way of the Edsel. Today management acknowledges its mistakes and corrects them quickly.

Trust is built step-by-step over a period of time. However, a major stride in reversing a climate of distrust can be effected by changing an untrustworthy behavior, followed by consistently engaging in *trust building* behavior. An actual experience will illustrate this point. A major grievance was settled without arbitration when management acknowledged it violated a provision of the contract. The grievance had to do with shift rotation. Although only two employees filed grievances, management recognized that making payments to just the employees who filed the grievance was unfair. Instead, the work records of every affected employee were evaluated and management voluntarily made payments to each of them, including those who had not openly complained. That good

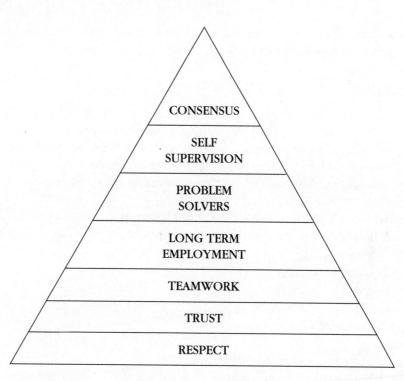

**FIGURE 7.1** Employee Empowerment

will enabled the organization to resolve several very difficult issues in subsequent contract negotiations.

## *Open Two-Way Communication*

Consistently woven in the fabric of any successful business or personal relationship is open, bi-directional communication; and this is level three. In the work environment, any number of forums can be developed and nurtured to encourage and improve effective communications. Focus group meetings or skip level meetings (skip level meetings are those held without the immediate manager) are a preliminary step in fostering open verbal exchanges. Print media are a very effective and powerful communication tool when the employee is the focus, or better yet, a contributor to the publication. Utilizing recorded messages on a "hot line" call-in is an efficient and useful means of disseminating important information. Employee-sponsored, "in-house" radio stations have a positive and sometimes humorous impact on communications. Any or all of these communication methods are relatively simple to initiate and maintain. Each has potential for a return on investment well beyond the cost of implementation.

## Teamwork

What the Japanese have demonstrated best is teamwork, which is the third level. The holistic view of the worker and his relationship to the organization goes back to Japan's rice-growing system. While one person working alone can not grow enough rice to feed a family, efforts combined with ten other families can feed more than fifty families. The Japanese dedication to teamwork is further evidenced in their avid support for a U.S. game, baseball.

Strangely, North Americans are good at team sports, but compete internally in the work place. If the goal is to hire and develop team players, the following must be evident of the candidate(s).

1. effective, open communicators
2. good listeners
3. supportive of others
4. genuinely respectful of others' views
5. trustworthy
6. seekers of agreement rather than dominance
7. loyal to other organization members
8. global thinkers who speak in terms of we, not I
9. willing to do menial tasks and projects

A first-hand experience demonstrates *all* of the above. While visiting a nursing facility, we asked to be introduced to the person in the institution who best exemplified team work. A small, frail, older adult woman was identified. It was her practice that whenever she finished her work she sought the persons who had the heaviest patient assignments and offered to do their most onerous tasks so that they could finish the remainder of their assignments. The outcome is obvious—everyone wanted her to work with them, and they all rushed to help her when she was overloaded with work.

## Long-Term Employment

Most often associated with the Japanese business environment is long-term employment; this is the fourth level in the pyramid. Recently, as a result of the economic downturn in Japan, there appears to be an erosion of their acclaimed commitment to lifetime employment. Although U.S. employers have not rushed to provide long-term work guarantees, the ample value of a stable work force has been recognized and rewarded in more contemporary health care systems. The cost of replacing a direct care nurse (registered nurse) at one hospital-based home health agency exceeds $43,000. This includes the cost of advertising, recruiting, temporary replacement, precepting, and so forth. It does not include the cost of disrupted patient care, loss of qualified professionals, lost productivity, or lost revenue.

Removing the threat of job loss for productive employees leads to new approaches for utilization of the work force. Employers who provide long-term employment realize the significant operational advantages from applying greater resources to improve the quality of their hiring, orientation, and training practices. The net result from hiring and investing in outstanding employees is multiplied by such employees' years of service. It is enhanced when marginal or nonproductive problem people are no longer considered for employment.

In Japanese companies, and American companies such as Wal-mart, employees are selected who share the organization's values and goals. Employees who are likely to stay and make an outstanding team contribution are the most valuable. Be skeptical of those with exceptional scholastic abilities and star quality resumes with five or ten different jobs in the last few years.

The March, 1990, issue of *HR Magazine* reported on the approach Toyota Motors used to staff its new plant in Kentucky. They recruited 60,000 applicants for 3,000 jobs (Costentino, Allen, & Wellins, 1990). They used a long and costly eight-step process that began with an orientation for every applicant. This orientation covered the company's values, philosophy, and expectations. It also included technical, interpersonal, and performance exercises, leadership assessments, teamwork simulations, group discussion, and problem-solving exercises. Toyota spent a great deal of time and money on an extremely well-planned and detailed recruiting process to get the kind of people who would stay with them, and work well within their system.

Once a stable work force has been hired, extensive and sometimes expensive educational programs can be instituted. Any organization is hesitant to invest time and money in an employee who suffers from "employment wanderlust." Montefiore Medical Center in the Bronx, New York, pioneered student loan programs for health care industry employees who wanted to train for market-scarce technical jobs. To earn loan forgiveness, the newly trained employee must work a fixed time period after completing school. The organization gains a long-term, loyal, committed employee while reducing recruiting costs *and* filling market-scarce positions.

Long-term employment in the U.S. work place can become a reality through better planning, better management, and the effective use of supplemental staff. The health care industry as a whole will have to adopt the successful techniques of other industries to be competitive as it faces health care reform.

## Employees as Problem Solvers

Problem-solving employees are on the fifth level. Success in an organization depends on expanding the jobs of all employees so they become data collectors, data analyzers, and problem solvers. A case in point—a New York area nursing home intended to make a change in food service by utilizing smaller patient meal trays. Before buying new carts, the dishwasher was asked for help in solving the problem. He suggested keeping the old carts and leaving the old trays in them as shelves, negating the need to purchase new carts. The nursing home saved $6,000 and the employee gained a sense of pride and ownership in the organization—a win/win outcome.

The evolving environment of managed care will dictate the employment of staff who are problem solvers. Economy and efficiency will be the survival tool of health care organizations. Monetary savings as described above may appear to be inconsequential, but when added together can be most impressive.

## Self Supervision

Nearly at the pinnacle of the pyramid is self supervision; it is a natural byproduct of the realization of the previous levels. The Japanese recognized that decision-making at the lowest level increased problem solving, effectiveness, and ultimately productivity. Also, people behave as adults when they supervise themselves, thus obviating the need for layers of staff and supervision. Self supervision permits more people to be available to perform the functions that actually produce a product or service. These efforts form the basis for a radically different approach toward implementing change.

## Planning and Consensus Building

The last level, and obviously the most lofty, is planning and consensus building. By using a time-consuming process of planning and consensus building, the Japanese are able to dramatically shorten implementation time. This may not seem to make sense, but the time spent in planning is offset by the time that would be consumed in troubleshooting and correcting mistakes *after implementation.* In contrast, after cursory planning, with little or no consensus building, employees in the U.S. rush headlong into projects. The end result may be that it takes longer to implement change, increases levels of frustration, inflates costs and, worst of all, becomes an out-and-out disaster. Health care organizations that are able to effect change efficiently and with the least amount of trauma will be in the best position to be successful in the coming era of health care reform.

The model of solving problems from the bottom up and building consensus using teams can pay off handsomely. It may take longer in the earlier stages, but projects are finished faster and with fewer problems. Once a work force is committed to teamwork and excellence, the institution begins moving toward long-term quality and productivity. While it may not always be possible to achieve consensus, the value it contributes toward bringing commitment from all who participate makes the effort worthwhile.

The art of management is changing around the world from the old authoritarian approach to a new and more effective way built on mutual respect, trust, communication, job security, teamwork, and consensus. In other cultures Americans are perceived as knowing no moderation, only extremes. In the past our business behavior has borne this statement out. In order to survive in a world economy and a vastly different health care economy, adoption of some traits, attitudes, and behaviors of the successful international market must be incorporated into American business practice. The remaining two segments of the triad, *improving patient care effectiveness* and *strategic patient service*, must be incorporated to make continuous quality improvement a reality.

# IMPROVING PATIENT CARE EFFECTIVENESS

The goal of improving patient care effectiveness is *eliminating waste so a greater amount of total available time and resources can be devoted to giving better care to more patients.* Goal achievement is realized by accomplishing four objectives.

1. Developing a culture of improvement. In this industry, that translates to improving the quality of all aspects of patient care service.
2. Eliminating waste. Maximization of all resources such as personnel, equipment, energy, and capital to reduce the cost per patient.
3. Continually reducing thruput time. Minimization of the amount of time it takes to deliver quality care.
4. Continually improving flexibility to respond to change.

If health care organizations are to survive in the coming era of reform, they must reduce, or better yet, eliminate the time spent on activities patients do not need or want. A home health care agency (HHA) must expand the amount of time spent providing care and simultaneously reduce the cost per visit.

How many times would a nurse be permitted to administer the wrong medication to a patient? How many times would a physical therapist be allowed to incorrectly teach crutch walking? How often can a pilot forget to engage the landing gear? The ability to achieve near-perfect quality depends on how important the task is to an individual or an organization, how costly it is to achieve, and how costly it is *not* to ensure quality.

Phil Crosby, a leading American quality expert, writes in his book *Quality is Free* that the cost of fixing mistakes is far greater than doing a task right the first time. The cost of malpractice insurance and the threat to professionals of loss of license make this cost ratio even greater. Quality experts claim 85 percent of quality errors are due to flaws in the system and not the fault of the individual worker. It is the responsibility of management to correct the flaws.

Some of the best techniques for quality improvement of patient care systems have already been tried and discarded. In the late 1970s and early 1980s, Americans thought *quality circles* alone were the secret weapon that was the key to Japanese success. When they did not take hold quickly and bring dramatic results, quality circles were abandoned. Utilization of some form of employee problem-solving teams and employee suggestion systems should be reconsidered. They can produce great results if integrated with a larger overall value system of continuous improvement and the other elements of the pyramid of excellence. The immense success of Toyota's Quality Circle approach of utilizing a work force committed to making meaningful contributions to team goals is most impressive. In 1960, Toyota averaged one suggestion per employee with one in ten being usable. By 1983, 38.5 suggestions per employee with a 95 percent acceptance rate had been realized (Cosentino, Allen, & Wellins, 1990). Toyota's results took two-plus decades to achieve, but what an achievement!

The second major Japanese contribution to quality improvement is *standardizing up.* They identify the last, best way something was done and teach everyone that method. It is based on the simple principle that tasks become easier to do as they are learned. Remember how hard it was to learn to drive a car and how easy it is to do now. Once a better way is learned, it becomes the new standard or foundation from which to launch the next series of improvements. The key is to avoid backward slippage once any level of improvement has been attained.

A typical problem solving model includes a five-step, commonsense approach.

1. Identify the problem
2. Identify the cause(s)
3. Identify the solution(s)
4. Evaluate the solution(s)
5. Select the best solution

However, in a quality, results-oriented organization, four important new steps are added.

**6. Standardize those improvements**
**7. Teach everyone the new method**
**8. Verify that the improvement actually works**
**9. Build in continuous improvement**

Initiating a standardize-up process provides limitless opportunity for sustained progress. Some may argue that this process works for making cars or television sets, but does not consider the uniqueness of the "people care" industry. Consider this analogy. The Japanese have mastered competitive auto sales in part because they applied the principle of standardizing up to what had previously been optional equipment on a car. By standardizing the most desirable options into their cars (those things that almost everyone wanted), they have improved quality, reduced cost, and made the customer's decision in the showroom easier: they standardized up. American car manufacturers have begun to embrace that system.

In a local nursing home, twenty-eight different models of wheelchairs were in use. Consider the potential savings in time, money, and even some better quality of care opportunities if only two or three models with the most commonly requested options were purchased. Maintenance would be easier, availability of the right chair in the right place at the right time would be realized, and purchasing advantages would probably be gained from dealing with fewer suppliers.

Many unique elements of patient care can not be standardized. However, that is no excuse for ducking the opportunities that exist for standardizing improvements in all the other areas that are not unique. Consider techniques like work flow analysis, clustering care givers in geographic areas, reducing interruptions, removing obstacles to speed thruput of the professional's paperwork, and reducing the time a care giver spends in the office. Positive actions to address just these few items would be beneficial to patients, staff, and the home care agency.

Both Japanese and American organizations are achieving greater flexibility by drastically reducing the number of job classifications and cross training people in multiskilled occupations. These employees are then paid more and utilized more effectively. An example of this is the emergence of the *rehabilitation nurse* in the home health care arena to augment the physical and occupational therapists. The rehabilitation nurse brings a new and expanded function to any rehabilitation service by reducing the need, or at least number, of skilled nursing visits required. The rehabilitation nurse is able to provide the necessary rehabilitation component *and* render the skilled nursing component. At the same time, the home health agency realizes economic savings by lowering the cost per patient served, gaining great improvements in flexibility, and providing career ladders or specialization for professional staff.

## STRATEGIC PATIENT SERVICES

The final component of the triad is *strategic patient service*. Patient service embraces all who are involved with the patient: family members, physicians, payers, hospitals, nursing homes, and the community.

Strategic patient service is dependent on

1. dedicating management to making patient service a strategic issue
2. hiring and educating a staff of super service employees
3. finding *all* complaints from *all* sources
4. promptly resolving identified complaints
5. developing systems to permanently remove the causes of patient and extended family dissatisfaction
6. instilling an attitude of global service rather than "it is not my job"

Super service begins with a management commitment to raise service to a strategic level for the entire organization. This concept of super service requires that each person acts as both a customer and a supplier of services. In order for an organization to develop habits of service excellence, it needs a disciplined commitment by all of its members to stay the course in meeting the organization's goals. Every employee must voluntarily commit and internalize the objectives and success of the organization to provide **outstanding** service—the service that sets your agency apart and above all others.

## CONCLUSION

Home health has a unique opportunity for service that no other segment of health care has; home care becomes part of the household and personnel may become surrogate family. Far too often, especially in the inner city, personnel from the HHA may be the only contact the patient has with the outside world.

Any organization that can bring the triad *humanizing the work place, improving patient care effectiveness,* and *strategic patient service* together will be successful in meeting the challenges of the coming reform in health care and solving the dichotomy of increasing demand and decreasing dollars. The challenge is great, but so are the rewards. Not moving toward the super service organization is also a great risk, and the penalties will be devastating to patients, professionals, and organizations.

"Empowered people are involved and committed to their work, and they gain satisfaction from their successes. For empowered individuals, caring for others and making the organization work better are two sides of the same coin. One cannot be achieved without the other" (Byham, 1993).

## REFERENCES

Byham, W. (1993). *Zapp! Empowerment in health care.* New York, NY: Fawcett Columbine.

Cosentino, C., Allen, J., & Wellins, R. (1990, March). Choosing the right people. *HR Magazine,* pp. 66–70.

Kolata, G. (1992, November 16). New views on life spans alter forecasts on elderly. *The New York Times,* pp. A1, A15.

## Suggested Readings

Fukuda, R. (1983). *Managerial engineering.* New York Productivity Press.

Schares, G. & Schwartz, E.I. (1992, November 16). Capitalism that would make Karl Marx proud. *Business Week,* pp. 82–83.

Schonberger, R. (1982). *Japanese manufacturing techniques.* New York: The Free Press.

Schulmerich, S.C. (1993). An analysis of job morale factors of community health nurses who report a low turnover rate; a nurse executive responds. *Journal of Nursing Administration,* 23(6), 27–28.

Taylor, J. (1983). *Shadows of the rising sun.* New York: William Marrow & Co. Inc.

# CHAPTER

8

# A Comprehensive Computer System for the Home Health Agency

**Ed Kahn**

Installation of a *comprehensive computer system* is one of the primary elements for survival and success in the coming era of managed care, capitation, and health care reform. A comprehensive computer system is defined as automating operations of multiple departments that rely on one another for completing a portion of the agency's work flow. It is not the individual use of personal computers for word processing or spreadsheets. Nationally marketed home care applications already exist, and include

- generic business functions (payroll, general ledger, and accounts payable)
- home health care business applications (Health Care Financing Administration [HCFA] form preparation, electronic and hard copy billing, and accounts receivable)
- clinical applications (patient assessments, physician orders, and chart notes)

Automation of an agency is a significant expense in *time and money*. A disastrous automation project leaves future automation projects questionable. Critical considerations and factors in implementing an automated home care system will be discussed in this chapter.

## BASIC PRINCIPLES FOR SUCCESSFUL COMPUTER PROJECTS

First and foremost, selecting, purchasing, installing, and making productive use of a computer system are an exercise in managing people's expectations. Continuous exposure to news, entertainment, and advertising creates unrealistic expectations of what computers are capable of doing.

The use of personal computers (PCs) has exploded in the last decade. However, PC literacy does not translate to an understanding of the installation of a major business application. Realizing the phenomena of unrealistic expectations at all levels of the organization is crucial.

In a home health care agency (HHA) unreasonable expectations can be especially acute among the clinically oriented staff. Their focus is delivering patient care. In general they view administrative chores as an unwelcome peripheral activity. Unfortunately, the more tried-and-true HHA applications automate administrative functions such as billing, in which clinical staff may take little interest. Installing a new computer system requires changes in administrative procedures, which may have significant impact on the clinical staff. As they climb the learning curve, clinical staff may even come to view the computer as something that *increases* their work. Their preinstallation expectations might have been that administrative tasks would be made easier, with little or no effort on their part. When perceived expectations and reality do not match, the result can lead to undesirable behavior and damage to the project.

Another class of future computer users with unreasonable expectations are those who readily admit to being afraid of computers, or so-called "computer-phobes." They can be a blessing in disguise. A computer-phobe can be defined as someone who is smart enough to know when they do not know something, and honest enough to share that fact. When handled properly, novice users can become the biggest success stories in a computer project, as they conquer fears and become more productive by employing newly acquired skills. Their success, when recognized and rewarded, can be made contagious, thus positively influencing others.

Two basic determinants of success in an automation project are management *commitment* to the project and users *desire* for the system.

Management commitment encompasses involvement of the senior manager in the following.

- obtaining necessary resources
- assigning appropriate project team members
- understanding the capabilities and limitations of available systems
- attending meetings and monitoring progress
- negotiating contracts
- recognizing and rewarding achievement

User desire for automation requires an honest appraisal of the willingness and inclination of affected staff to be *change agents*. A committed internal sponsor, or informal leader, is an invaluable asset for successful implementation. Identifying the internal sponsor(s) is one of the first tasks of management.

## The Project and Project Team

Since managing expectations is the key to success in automation, a context within which to manage expectations must be produced. This context is provided by recognizing that successfully selecting, purchasing, and installing a computer system is a *project* that will be completed by a *project team*.

# THE PROJECT

A *project* is a unit of work that has a defined beginning, a defined end, and clearly defined objectives. The *project team* is the vehicle through which the project is accomplished.

The objectives of a project must be measurable. Measurable objectives serve to focus project efforts on the overall outcome, and provide the means to assess the success of the effort.

Because a project has a defined lifetime that can span many months, it is convenient to manage a project in *phases* that comprise the project's life cycle. The phases represent periods of activity directed toward production of an *interim product*. The interim product is a document that records the result of the work performed during each phase and marks the milestone that evidences the end of each phase. Milestone documentation enables management to monitor progress and endorse proceeding to the next phase; it also provides continuity should team personnel change during the life of the project.

Milestone documentation can alert management to problems at the earliest possible time, as well, avoiding unnecessary expenditures on work that will need to be redone.

For a significant automation project, the following project phases are usually appropriate.

- formation
- evaluation
- detailed design
- implementation
- postimplementation review

Each phase represents an increase in the organizational learning that has been accomplished. In the first phase, only sketchy information is available, and is coarse and lacking many details. As the project proceeds through the phases, details are fleshed in and pinned down. Table 8.1 summarizes major project management phases.

## Formation Phase

The formation phase allows management to determine if a business problem exists that automation is likely to solve within a reasonable time and for acceptable cost. The tasks of the formation phase are to

- describe the business problem that automation is likely to solve
- identify the objectives for the project
- identify the scope of the project
- identify and charter the project team

In the formation phase, relatively little detailed information is known about costs and benefits of automation; rather, the objective is to determine if it is *reasonably likely* that a detailed study would show significantly greater benefits than costs.

The document that marks the end of the formation phase is the *formation report*, which is an internal proposal for an automation project. It should discuss and analyze the business problem and its potential solution in general terms. It is appropriate to include data indicating the scope of operations to be affected and a general survey of possible alternative solutions.

Defining the scope and objectives of the project can be difficult. Consider what elements are absolutely critical for the success of the project and the organization. How much is too much for the scope of the project? Be wary of attempting more than can be completed in six to nine months. Automation projects are complex and can easily be bogged down if too much is undertaken. If the proposed project will take longer than six to nine months, it is probably better to divide the effort into multiple subprojects to be run sequentially, or concurrently if resources permit.

For instance, billing may currently be done manually, and as census grows, installation of an automated billing system will allow billing to be done more rapidly and accurately, without increasing staff. The formation phase of a project to procure and install

**TABLE 8.1** Overview of Project Life Cycle

| Phase | Formation | Evaluation | Design | Implementation | Postimplementation Review |
|---|---|---|---|---|---|
| Answers the questions: | What is the problem? Do we have a project? | Is the project worth doing? | How will we complete the project? | Did we solve the problem? | How can we do the next project better? |
| Attributes | Informal<br><br>Little invested, not much to lose. | Formal<br><br>Analyze alternatives<br><br>Assess feasibilities | Formal<br><br>Design specifications<br><br>Vendor selection | Formal<br><br>Tracked closely against the implementation plan developed in the Design Phase | Informal |
| Milestone Document | Formation report | Project evaluation report | Vendor contract<br><br>Implementation plan | Users' acceptance of implemented system | Postimplementation review report |
| Duration | Short 1–10 days | 20%–30% of total project<br><br>Typically 1–2 months | 30%–50% of total project<br><br>Typically 2–4 months | 25%–35% of total project<br><br>Typically 1–3 months | Short 1–2 days |

an automated billing system would document the census growth, labor, and other costs of manual billing, the time it takes to bill, the error rate (based on sampling), the collection rate, and how long it takes to collect. It would then estimate the impact installing an automated system would have on these parameters. This impact estimate describes and quantifies, where possible, the expected benefits. The formation phase could also identify available home care billing systems and estimate the costs of procuring, installing, and operating them.

A comprehensive billing system has information links to accounts receivable and general ledger. In scoping this project, a question needs to be asked and answered. Can an integrated billing and accounts receivable system be installed in approximately the same amount of time as a stand-alone billing system? If not, is it worth the extra cost and effort?

In addition to sketching the business problem to be solved and its possible solutions, the formation report should identify a proposed project team and a plan for the next phase, or *evaluation.*

The formation phase should not take a long time. One to ten working days should suffice. Remember, in formation, develop only enough detail to convince management that an automation project is likely to be beneficial, and which among the possible projects is likely to be most beneficial.

To the extent that existing staff lacks experience in the process of implementing an automation project, consider investing in outside expertise to assist in the formation phase. Hiring a consultant who practices primarily in HHAs, has knowledge of the industry and available vendors' offerings, and has experience assisting agencies in scoping automation projects can be a cost-effective way to complete a formation phase and resulting formation report.

### The Project Manager and Project Team

Once management has reviewed and accepted the formation report, the project team must be identified. A project team is led by a *project manager* who is responsible for planning and allocating resources, assigning and tracking tasks, conducting team meetings, and reporting to management.

The choice of a project manager is very important. A qualified project manager must be a leader, teacher, administrator, and coach. The project manager must inspire confidence and be able to communicate with a broad spectrum of personnel who work in the agency—from senior management, clinical staff, clerical workers, and those outside the agency such as potential vendors, their present customers, and attorneys for both sides.

The project manager must possess the ability to detect when expectations of people participating in the project are not in line with reality, and take appropriate steps to correct the situation. This ability is crucial because the clues that expectations are out of line can be subtle, and the range of remedial actions is broad—education, reorganization, rewards, and so forth.

If the project manager lacks these skills, the administrator must be prepared to spend time engaged in the project to compensate. If this necessary work is left improperly staffed, the project will most assuredly fail.

Since the project has a defined beginning and end, it is possible to staff the project manager position with an outside consultant specialist, preferably one with a track record of successfully implementing similar automation projects in the home health industry. The remainder of the project team should be composed of people from the areas to be affected. Ideal project team members are natural leaders from their respective areas who are eager to "change things for the better." Since this will entail extra work on the part of those who already may view themselves as overburdened, it is important that assignment to the project team be viewed as special and important, both of which are *true.* The feeling of importance must remain fresh within the project team for the duration of the project. Senior managers may find that this responsibility is perhaps their most important task.

The ground rules must be clear when chartering the project team. One important rule is that meeting notes be kept and circulated to team members. The notes will document discussions and decisions made by the project team. This helps keep team members and management current on project progress. Additionally, it provides continuity and consistency to project activities, even if staff should change as the project proceeds.

## Evaluation Phase

The evaluation phase begins when management determines that the formation report has made a case for investing in a detailed investigation of alternatives to solve a recognized business problem.

The purpose of the evaluation phase is to achieve a fairly detailed understanding of options available to solve the identified business problem and determine the costs and benefits of automation. Roughly a quarter of the entire project is spent in this phase.

The *evaluation report,* often called a "cost/benefit analysis," is the product of the evaluation phase. This report should be detailed enough to enable management to choose from the available alternatives for *this* project. Typically, alternatives include one or more "packaged" vendor systems, development of a customized system to meet the agency's individual and *unique* specifications, or the purchase of "shared services" through a service bureau. Each of these alternatives will present different costs and benefits, which the evaluation report must analyze. Figure 8.1, outlines the typical sections.

In order to accomplish the evaluation phase, the project team will require education in two general areas of agency operation. First, how does the agency currently operate in the areas proposed for automation and what capabilities will be required in a system to solve the business problem identified in the formation report? Second, what alternative systems are available that provide the functionality needed in those areas, and what will be the impact of each?

The project team must study and document the present system. In the areas to be affected, who does what, when, and how? There are many methodologies and tools for accomplishing this; an experienced project manager has likely adopted favorite tools and techniques. For detailed information on the topic of methodologies, references are cited at the conclusion of the chapter. An HHA automation project is usually not large and intricate enough to justify the expense of strict adherence to a particular formal methodology and tool set for describing the present system and its information flows. While it may be advantageous, it is not a prerequisite.

### The Current System

Information about the current system is documented by interviewing the people who participate in operating the system, and recording what is learned. It consists of meeting

Table of Contents
Definition of the Business Problem
    Purpose and Objectives
    Current Operations in the Affected Business Units
    Proposed Systems and Operations in the Affected Business Units
Data, Technical and Operational Feasibility
    Equipment Considerations
    Service and Operating Considerations
    Sources of Data
Alternatives
    Findings
    Recommendations
    Development Plan
Estimated Costs
    Initial Cost Analysis
    Recurring Cost Analysis
Payback
    Cash Flow
    Economic Feasibility
    Intangible benefits
Attachments

**FIGURE 8.1** Outline of Project Evaluation Report

notes, process flowcharts, budgets, operating indicators, and other data tables collected and collated by the project team. This is a voyage of agency self-discovery, and it can have impressive, unexpected benefits. It may also be painful.

During the process of discovery, more than once project team members will exclaim, "I never knew we did that!" Additionally, structured self-examination is an opportunity to engender feelings of ownership in the soon-to-be installed computer system. The net result will be a renewed sense of confidence among staff who, by their participation in the evaluation process, buy into the results.

In the evaluation phase, the project team will prepare a list of requirements the system must fulfill. These are divided into two general classes: functional requirements and performance requirements. Functional requirements state what the new computer system must do. For example, a billing system must produce bills in the formats required by payers. Performance requirements identify the volumes of work the proposed system will have to process in a defined time frame. For instance, an on-line system interacts with its users via terminals to process transactions one at a time, and must perform quickly enough to avoid keeping the user waiting. A performance requirement might be an $X$ second response time.

By dissecting the present system, the picture of what will change and the functionality needed to change it will be clearer, and it will be easier to evaluate alternatives. At this point alternative solutions can be considered.

## Alternative Systems

Identification and analysis of potential solutions are next in the process. However, potential solution investigation can proceed in parallel with documenting the present system and proposed system requirements. Potentially promising systems will have been listed during the formation phase, and investigation into these systems can begin as requirements are being clarified.

There are a number of valuable sources for locating potential solutions. National, regional, and state meetings are well-attended by vendors, whose booth displays can introduce systems being offered. Advertising appearing in trade publications is another source. Contacting agencies that resemble your agency and inquiring how they handle similar problems and situations can produce volumes of valuable information. These efforts should produce a list of potential solutions and the vendors that provide them.

Once interest is expressed to a potential vendor, the agency will become a target of their sales effort. The project team should utilize this energy to become educated about what the vendor's system does, how well it works in other customer locations, and what the experience of being this vendor's customer has been.

Potential vendors should be invited to make presentations to the project team. The presentation can be repeated until the team has a good sense of what the vendor claims the system can do. The project team should also inspect the vendor's written user documentation (manuals). These should be logically organized and clearly written. Since a new computer system will introduce many new terms, look for definitions. Definitions should make new concepts clear *before* someone has to use these concepts to understand new material.

Concurrently, the vendor should identify other similar clients and arrange for them to act as references. In addition to talking in depth with these references, selected members of the project team should make site visits to a representative sample. At some point during the site visit, the vendor should leave so that candid dialogue between the actual and potential customer can take place. Be suspicious if the vendor is reluctant to accommodate the request to talk or visit with its client without a representative being present.

One important decision the organization must make is how formal a process to follow in selecting a vendor and negotiating a contract. This is largely dictated by the scope of the project; the larger the project and the more alternatives there are to choose from, the more formal a process should be followed.

***Request for Information.*** During the investigation into potential vendors, many questions will need to be asked and answered. To develop a "standard" set of responses from multiple vendors, issuing a request for information (RFI) is appropriate. This document, prepared by the project team during the evaluation phase, consists of two sections.

◈

1. *Information about the agency.* In this section, the potential vendor becomes acquainted with the agency and what the expectations are for a system. This enables the vendor to demonstrate aspects of the system that will be most meaningful and effectively address needs.

2. *Agency system requirements.* System expectations are enumerated in this section. The vendor is asked to respond, point by point, to how the system accomplishes or fails to accomplish each item. System requirements expressed in measurable terms enable the team to compare vendors' responses.

***Costs to be Investigated.*** The RFI should ask the vendors to propose a hardware and software configuration to meet stated requirements. Require the vendor to specify unit costs of anything to be bought in multiples, such as terminals. In addition, recurring costs like software maintenance fees, telephone charges, etc., must be identified. Typical costs to be investigated include

- hardware—the computer and attached equipment such as terminals, printers, tape drives, disk drives, and so forth
- operating system software—the computer program(s) that enable the vendor's application to communicate with and make use of the hardware
- application software—the computer program(s) the vendor provides to meet your business requirements
- communications hardware—modems, control units, interface boards, patch panels, and any other items needed to provide remote access to the system
- cabling—signal cable, terminators, and labor needed to link hardware and communications hardware together
- maintenance and enhancements—service when something "breaks," which includes program bugs, hardware failure, and communications outages. Enhancements include provision of new programs when the requirements the system is designed to meet have changed, such as when HCFA requires a new or redefined field on a bill. Additional enhancements may result when multiple users identify a common need.
- site preparation—power, uninterruptible power supply (UPS), air-conditioning, physical security, measures to deal with disaster recovery (flood or fire)
- conversion—inputting manual records and/or reformatting already computerized records for use by the new system. Often these two need to be merged after differences between them have been reconciled.
- customization—programs to be added to the system to meet unique needs of the agency. How will charges be incurred—time and materials, or by the job?
- interfaces—programs to be written to link this system to other systems used by the agency, hospital, or parent organization
- installation—labor and materials needed to uncrate and set up hardware, and load and test software
- training—initial and ongoing education of staff in the use of the system

- service—if the hardware is manufactured by an organization other than the software provider (this is most likely the case), then the agency should insist on "one-stop shopping." In other words, if something "goes wrong," only one phone call to the software vendor is necessary to obtain service, irrespective of whether the problem is in the hardware or software.

**Vendor Evaluation.**   Deal formally with potential vendors in the RFI process. Conduct a meeting for all interested vendors so they will clearly understand agency requirements prior to submission of responses. Set a concrete deadline for response submission with a strict requirement for adherence to format. A great deal of difficulty comparing responses among vendors will result if format is not followed. Format adherence also reduces the likelihood of "boilerplate" responses.

Evaluating vendor responses presents a real challenge. Purchasing, installing, and using a comprehensive system is a complex process; responses could be scored using a variety of methodologies. However, subjectivity may be the "rule of thumb" rather than the exception. The purpose of the detailed RFI is to bring *facts* to light about what a proposed system does and how it performs; whether a particular system is *right* for your organization is determined by far more than just the facts presented.

It may be useful to "score" the RFI responses by applying relative weights to the questions in the RFI, and numerical values to the answers. Scoring consists of multiplying the questions' weights by their answers' values and tabulating the results. The alternative with the highest score should represent the best alternative. But be careful. Use this methodology only if you are convinced that scoring will justify the work of designing and agreeing upon the weights, scores, and methodology within the project team. Usually, this technique is needed only when the project team is unable to reach a consensus and needs to make the choice more objective.

The useful life of a comprehensive system is at least five years. But the agency may be living with the system for ten, fifteen, or even twenty years. The proposed system must continue to meet critical requirements and perform to reasonable expectations over this long time span. Therefore, the system should provide an evolution path as business changes with time. For example, if visit volume increases significantly, the proposed system must provide an upgrade path that avoids the need to convert to a new system. In other words, the proposed application should run *unchanged* on bigger, faster hardware as it becomes available.

**Interfaces.**   If new related lines of business are on the horizon for the agency, consider whether the system proposed by the vendor also supports the new business line(s). Interfacing foreign systems, where one vendor's system supports one business line and another vendor's system supports another business line, is very risky. Try to avoid interfaces unless there is a substantial track record of successful installations of identical interfaces among current clients of these vendors. Even if an interface appears to be usable without modifications, there are many opportunities for trouble in which each vendor blames the other's side of the interface or the other's application. By keeping from interfaces, the agency avoids a potentially crippling malfunction and being caught in a tug-of-war between competing vendors.

Unfortunately, interfaces cannot always be avoided. When the need for an interface outweighs the risk, proceed cautiously. In the *detailed design* phase, pay attention to what might change over the system's lifetime that would affect the interface, and provide for these in the contract negotiations. In the section "Contract Negotiations," this will be discussed.

***Packaged Systems.*** Much of what has already been discussed applies primarily to obtaining a "packaged" system. A packaged system consists of a core set of computer program(s) a vendor offers to multiple similar businesses who use that programming without making changes to it. In designing a packaged system, the vendor attempts to anticipate differences in the ways potential users will need to use the system, and provides functions within the system for these idiosyncrasies.

No vendor can do a perfect job of anticipating the needs of all potential clients, so there will be elements of any packaged system that will be awkward to use, or simply not required to meet the agency's needs.

***Customized Systems.*** The primary alternative available for addressing deficiencies in a packaged system is custom development; this is computer programming develops specifically for the agency's needs. In the most extreme case, there may be no packaged system that addresses the needs of the agency and thus an entire system must be custom developed. This is unlikely in the home health industry, where packaged systems are available to support much of the core business function. Avoid custom development unless a unique system would provide a strategic advantage and funding is not a constraint.

***Advantage of Phased Approach.*** One of the advantages of employing a phased approach is the opportunity to assess the validity of continuing the project at defined checkpoints. As evaluation proceeds, it may be discovered that modifications to manual procedures or limited assistance from a computer service bureau will meet agency needs and deliver most of the benefits thought achievable only by using an in-house system. This could be a significant triumph because it enables improvement in operations without a large investment.

Most likely, evaluation will show one or a small number of reasonable alternative vendor systems where benefits exceed the costs. During evaluation the project team will have formed opinions on which system and which vendor is preferred, derived in part from the objective information produced by the RFI, and in part by subjective impressions garnered in interaction with the vendor's personnel and clients during site visits. Any preference should be concealed from the vendor at this time, lest negotiating leverage be lost.

Management review and approval of the evaluation report bring the evaluation phase to a close, and authorize proceeding to the detailed design phase.

# DETAILED DESIGN PHASE

The purpose of the detailed design phase is to produce a blueprint for the completion of the project and a plan for implementation. The objective of the design phase is to specify *what* computer system will be implemented, *who* will implement it, *when* implementation will be complete, and *how much,* within five to ten percent, it will cost. In this phase, contracts will be negotiated with competing vendors, leading to vendor selection and contract signing. Additionally, a comprehensive plan will be developed for the implementation of the system.

## Detailed Design Specifications

The project team will produce the *detailed design specification,* which is the product of the design phase. Detail design specifications include

- the contract with the proposed system vendor(s) for procuring hardware, software, maintenance and enhancement services, custom programming costs, and hardware and software installation fees
- itemization of program specifications for interfaces and conversions that will be custom developed. These consist of detailed descriptions of program logic, file layouts, and report layouts.
- written operating procedures for each kind of user, describing when and how the user is to interact with the system
- new forms for collection of input. Controls for assuring all input is collected and processed correctly and in a timely manner.
- modification of existing job descriptions and creation of new ones necessitated by the installation of the system
- a written test plan that specifies a test for every important function in the system, and the expected outcome of each test. It should also specify who will be responsible for conducting the test, and when.
- construction or renovation plans, and any contracts needed for providing space and utilities for computer equipment and users. Typically included are electricity, telephone, climate conditioning, physical security, fire or flood protection, signal cabling, furniture, and decorating.
- a written training plan identifying learning objectives, who will receive what training, who will provide what training, and when
- a plan to disseminate information to all staff regarding the "new era." This is particularly important for staff who were not part of the project team.
- a routine downtime plan. This plan details the steps to be taken for routine or temporary (brief) periods when the system will not be available to end users. Routine downtime includes backups, monthly close processing, or when a component, for example, a hard disk drive, fails and requires repair or replacement. Typically, for brief outages (a few hours to a few days), the organization will have manual

procedures to fall back on. For example, data will be collected on forms, which will be input to the computer system once service is restored.

- an emergency plan. This details how backups will be taken and stored, and how to employ them if some catastrophe befalls the computer system. Depending on how critical availability of the system is, maintaining a redundant remote site could be considered. Fortunately, HHA applications are not typically so critical in nature, and thankfully so, because redundancy and instant availability are *very* expensive. The emergency plan needs to clarify how to continue agency operations for days or weeks, which usually means returning to a manual system. The plan will address where backup copies of information are stored in order to load a replacement computer to resume operations. *Off site* storage of backups prevents loss of agency data in the event of destruction of the agency office; it does not do much good to make backups that are destroyed in the same fire that melts the computers.

- a conversion plan. This identifies how to capture the initial "load" of information to start the new system going. This may involve writing a computer program(s) to capture already automated data from a predecessor system, or collecting paper records in batches and quickly inputting them into the computer system during a narrow conversion time frame just prior to live operation of the new system. If paper record processing will be necessary, batching will provide *batch control,* a means of cross-checking that all information was entered, and entered correctly, prior to starting live operations.

## Management of the Detailed Design Phase

The project team must accomplish a great deal of work during the detailed design phase. Do not forget that the organization is aware that major changes are coming, and their expectations require continuous attention. Managing change, especially the magnitude of an integrated automation project, requires volumes of bidirectional and lateral communication between management and staff. According to Duck (1993), "The crucial lesson here is that management is the message. Everything managers say—or don't say—delivers a message. Too many managers assume that communications is a staff function, something for human resources or public relations to take care of. In fact, communications must be a priority for every manager at every level of the company. This is particularly true during a change effort, when rumors run rampant. It is important for the messages to be consistent, clear, and endlessly repeated. If there is a single rule of communications for leaders, it is this: when you are so sick of talking about something that you can hardly stand it, your message is finally starting to get through."

Approximately one-third of the total project time is consumed in detailed design. Because of the many tasks the project team is trying to accomplish during this phase, it is easy for project team members to assign low priority to communicating with the rest of the organization. Do not let this happen. Hold meetings with staff throughout the organization and keep them informed about the project's progress. Welcome questions and suggestions. Publish a newsletter. Do whatever it takes to keep the entire organization current with developments regarding the work-in-progress. At best, the organization will develop a sense of enthusiasm and welcome the coming change, and at worst, will be able to adjust in an acceptable manner.

## Contract Negotiations

Negotiating an acceptable contract with the proposed system vendor begins the detailed design phase. Vendors will offer their standard agreement, which, as expected, is written to protect them, not the agency. While a comprehensive treatment of how to negotiate a contract is beyond the scope of this work, the dynamics of striking a bargain will be determined by the relative strength of the agency's desire to acquire the vendor's system versus the vendor's desire to have the agency as their client.

The contract should *detail* the rights and responsibilities of each party. This is extremely important because the written agreement will be referred to over the useful life of the system to ensure both parties live up their respective responsibilities. If a serious dispute arises with the vendor, the quality of the agreement will determine the outcome. Poorly worded, incomplete agreements lead to unpredictable outcomes, and the agency could be left without recourse. Obviously, the agreement is executed *before* installation.

The essence of the bargain is: the vendor will sell something, and will be paid for it. There are risks on both sides of this equation, and the purpose of the agreement is to anticipate and provide for them.

The first critical question is, what is the vendor selling? The vendor is likely to be selling a combination of things.

- hardware such as mainframes or personal computers, terminals, printers, communications gear, etc.
- operating system software (e.g., NETWARE, UNIX, MS-DOS, compilers)
- "packaged" application software such as billing and accounts receivable computer programs, a word processor, spreadsheet, etc.
- custom-developed software such as an interface to another computer system, or modifications to the vendor's packaged software to meet the agency's special needs
- services such as software installation and configuration, training, equipment setup, and maintenance
- supplies

Everything the vendor will sell must be completely and accurately described in the agreement. This is easy for discrete, tangible items such as computers, PCs, terminals, word processing packages, but more difficult for less tangible items like services and custom software development.

A primary concern for the agency will be that the vendor has the right to sell what is to be bought. Computer software is intellectual property, and intellectual property rights have been an actively developing area of law over the past few years. It would be an unpleasant surprise if a third party sued for unauthorized or unlicensed use of their alleged property.

In the agreement, the vendor should warrant they own or have the right to sell everything being sold, and provide a procedure for dealing with challenges to the vendor's rights. A typical provision is that the vendor will indemnify the agency against third-party claims, if the vendor is allowed to control the defense against the claim.

Price is certainly a negotiable item, and the agency can and should challenge the prices the vendor proposes. What is the *best price?* The best price is one that allows the vendor enough revenue to earn a *fair* return while providing the quality service expected. Challenge the vendor to justify proposed pricing to this standard.

Timing is critical to both parties. The agency wants the system installed according to an installation plan, *and* the system has to be usable to achieve its benefits. The vendor wants to deposit agency payments as soon as possible. This is a fertile area for negotiation!

### Custom Programming

Risk is what makes timing unpredictable, and the riskiest element of any computer system agreement is custom development. Historically, vendors have made many miscalculations of their own capabilities and customer expectations when developing custom software.

Vendor claims in the area of customization need to be put to the test. Is the vendor prepared to risk paying penalties for failure to deliver custom software or any other component on time? If not, what security will the agency have that the vendor can deliver on time? Do not allow the agency to be the only "risk taker" when it comes to custom programming. Each partner of the contract must assume some jeopardy in the custom program arena.

## Additional Contract Negotiation Considerations

The agency needs assurance that the vendor's system will provide service that meets a defined quality standard. The agreement must spell out what is meant by "quality service." A warranty provision in the agreement will define this. Typically, *performance, capacity, and service standards* will be delineated.

Performance standards express how quickly the computer system will be able to complete a unit of work. For example, interactive transactions must finish quickly enough so that a person interacting with the computer system will not be forced to wait. These kinds of transactions should not delay the human operator for more than a second or two. Another example: month-end, high-volume processes (such as monthly closings) and routine but vital maintenance (such as backups) must be completed in an acceptable amount of time, and not prevent routine use of the system while being performed.

A performance standard is important because it prevents the vendor from "lowballing," or selling less computer power than is actually needed in order to appear to have the most attractive price. To be worth something, the performance standard must have teeth. For example, the vendor could be required, at their expense and within a specified time frame, to upgrade the computer to meet the warranted performance.

Capacity standards describe how much data the computer will hold and still meet the performance standards. The amount of data any computer system can maintain on-line is finite. The agency must identify how much history is needed "on-line" to meet operational demand. Also, computer systems are designed with inherent limits. The vendor must certify that agency requirements do *not* approach design limits. For example, the agency patient identifier may be nine characters long and the computer system is designed to handle a maximum of eight characters, or the design of the system limits the number of concurrently active patients to some number below the usual or occasional census.

Anticipated changes in business over the expected useful life of the system must be addressed. If, for example, it is projected that volume will increase dramatically, try to obtain a warranty that the system will handle the increased volume, *and* will do so without degrading performance.

Service standards describe what responses the vendor will warrant when something appears broken. This is very important, particularly when a comprehensive system has been purchased from a vendor who has integrated their software with a number of components from third parties. When something appears broken, the primary vendor should be responsible for diagnosis and repair, even though the actual service may be provided by third parties. If service standards are not well-defined and agreed to *before* implementation, the agency will likely end up in the middle of a situation where all suppliers disclaim responsibility for the problem and the system remains broken.

Typically, a service warranty defines the maximum time allowed for a reported problem to be diagnosed and repaired. Additionally, it provides procedures for prioritizing problems with large impact ahead of problems with lesser impact.

A service warranty is difficult to enforce because failure to strictly live up to the letter of the agreement is usually not sufficient grounds for breaking the agreement. It usually means there are unnecessary annoyances in using the system, not that the system is totally unusable.

To prevent truly horrible service, the agreement should provide that a material breach of any of the standards will be grounds to break the agreement and impose substantial financial penalties on the vendor. Incorporate in this clause a provision stating that all of the data processed by the system are the agency's property and delineating the procedures by which the agency is entitled to migrate off of the vendor's system.

## Source Codes

The original computer programming, or *source code,* is not what is generally acquired when a system is purchased. What has been bought is a license to use the vendor's computer programming, without actually owning it. If the vendor enters bankruptcy, or assigns the rights to their application software to a third party, the agency's right to continue using the application could be called into question. To protect against this, an escrow provision should be included in the agreement. This generally provides for a copy of the source code to be placed in escrow with an independent third party, such as a bank, and released if the vendor enters bankruptcy or assigns their rights. It would be advantageous to have the escrow release triggered if the "right to cancel for cause" clause is invoked by the agency. Right to cancel could be invoked if the system did not meet performance, capacity, or service standards described above.

Obviously, a contract for a comprehensive computer system is a specialized, complicated instrument. An attorney familiar with computer systems agreements and intellectual property rights should, at a minimum, review any agreement *before* it is signed.

## System Acceptance

Approval of anything the vendor delivers must be conditional on the delivery passing an acceptance test. For hardware, this generally means the equipment will successfully process set-up diagnostic tests provided by the hardware manufacturer. For applications software and custom development, both parties, during negotiations, will agree on the tests the application will have to pass. Test cases with sets of sample input and the output expected from the system will be prepared by the agency. Before the agency will be obligated to pay for what has been delivered, the tests must be "passed." This area should be stated in the agreement.

Timing of payments will have been negotiated in the agreement. Agency strategy will be to delay payments until it is satisfied that what has been received is what was expected, *and negotiated.* Payments are the primary leverage the agency will have to get the vendor to correct system deficiencies in a timely manner.

While the contract is being negotiated, and for the remainder of the design phase, the project team will attend to elements such as written operating procedures for users, new forms for collection of data, and so forth, all of which have been identified earlier in this section. Once management reviews and approves, the project can enter the next phase, implementation.

# IMPLEMENTATION PHASE

The purpose of the *implementation phase* is to execute the installation, training, testing, and conversion plans developed in the detail design phase. The primary tasks of the implementation phase are to pay close attention to progress vis-à-vis the implementation plans and keep the staff involved and informed as implementation progresses.

If there has been sufficient investment in time and effort during detail design, the implementation phase should proceed smoothly and predictably. If unforeseen problems or variances from the plan arise, early detection and immediate correction and/or modification are essential.

Testing is a critical activity during implementation. In previous phases, the project team will have designed test scripts and predicted results using agency data and processing requirements. The contract should have a clause defining what tests the newly installed system must pass for acceptance. Payment should hinge on the system passing. Payment may be partial as major components such as hardware, system software, and major pieces of application functionality meet acceptance criteria.

## User Education

User education should occur as close in time as possible to when the learned skills will be utilized with the new system. The success of education should be evaluated to determine if staff members who will be interactive with the system are ready to assume their new duties.

If remediation is necessary, do not simply repeat the training. This is like shouting and repeating in an attempt to make a foreign-speaking person understand when clearly she or he did not understand the language. It does not work, and encourages both parties to break off the interaction. Instead, diagnose the problem and try to understand why training was not successful the first time. Listen to the trainee and try a new approach.

## Making the System a Reality

Proper testing and the need to rework some processes brought to light by testing are time-consuming. Allow approximately one-third of the total project time for implementation.

During implementation many of the changes the system will bring become visible to staff who were not part of the project team. Space is renovated, hardware is delivered, cables are run, and so forth. As significant milestones occur, note them with special notices, celebrations, or acknowledgements. Hold a party in the "new" computer room. Ceremonially retire the old system. Recognize achievements as staff learn and employ new skills. Keep the staff excited and informed as progress is made.

No major implementation proceeds exactly as planned, but by following project management methodology and paying close attention to the expectations of the entire organization, chances of success will be maximized, and problems will be minimized during implementation and beyond. The agency will have put in the best system available to meet its unique requirements, and at the most reasonable cost.

# POSTIMPLEMENTATION REVIEW

After the system has been running for about six months, operations have stabilized to normal, and the effects of the new system are apparent, a postimplementation review should be conducted. The project team reconvenes and honestly appraises the outcome of the project against the objectives developed during the evaluation phase. Are the expected benefits flowing? Were the costs in line with expectations? How could the project have been improved?

A postimplementation review should take several hours to several days, at most. Taking the time and trouble to conduct postimplementation review will help the organization learn from the experience of having effected a major change, and will make the next project easier and more productive.

# CONCLUSION

An overview of the process of selecting and installing a comprehensive computer system for a home health agency has been presented. Computerizing operations requires changing attitudes and behaviors throughout the agency. This change process requires commitment and attention by the senior managers. Keeping staff informed and involved, and rewarding desired changes as they occur are key techniques to accomplish these difficult ends.

Selecting and installing a system is a project that will be accomplished over a defined time span, generally not longer than six to nine months. To make sure that the large investment in time, effort, and money is not wasted, it is vital to employ a project management methodology to plan and track the effort. The multiphase methodology discussed will enable the agency to assure that the computer system meets the identified needs at an affordable cost.

Wise managers know when to seek outside assistance. Such is the case in engaging consultants to supplement the agency staff in project management and contract negotiations.

A project of this scope will succeed to the extent that the agency understands what is needed and to what extent the vendor's system will meet those needs. The contract for the system *must be* a negotiated written agreement that expresses, in detail, the agency's needs and how the vendor will meet them. Key areas for negotiation have been offered; do not rely on the vendor's "standard" agreement.

The agency will maximize the benefits of its investment in selecting and installing a comprehensive computer system when the project is organized and implemented in a logical and measurable manner.

# REFERENCES

Duck, J.D. (1993). Managing change: The art of balancing. *Harvard Business Review,* pp. 109–118.

# *Suggested Readings*

Adams, D.A., & Mensching, J.R. (1991). *Managing an information system.* Englewood Cliffs, NJ: Prentice Hall.

Arnell, A. (1990). *Handbook of effective disaster/recovery planning.* New York: McGraw Hill.

Bisak, J. (1994). Leveraging information technology for business value. *The Remington report.* June/July, pp. 36–37.

Calhoun, Z. (1994). Five key strategies for selecting the right information system. *The Remington report.* June/July, pp. 39–41.

Computer Science and Telecommunications Board, National Research Council. (1991). *Intellectual property issues in software.* Washington, D.C.: National Academy Press.

Conner, D.R. (1993). *Managing at the speed of change.* New York: Villard Books.

Ince, D., Sharp, H. & Woodman, M. (1993). *Introduction to software project management and quality assurance.* New York: McGraw Hill Book Company Europe.

Lucas, H.C. Jr. (1992). *The analysis, design and implementation of information systems* 4th ed. New York: Mitchell McGraw Hill.

Quick, T.L. (1992). *Successful team building.* New York: AMACOM Division of the American Management Association.

Tanguay, P. (1994). Successful information system implementation. *The Remington Report.* June/July, pp. 13–15.

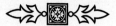

# PART TWO

## FINANCIAL MANAGEMENT

# CHAPTER

# Financial Requirements of a Home Health Agency

**Timothy Riordan**

As in all other types of businesses, the financial operation of a home health agency (HHA) requires general accounting and financial knowledge. Unlike any other business, specialized third-party reimbursement experience is necessary for fiscally sound management of an HHA. The home health environment has evolved dramatically in the past ten years. Total volume of visits has increased significantly. In addition to skilled nursing, rehabilitation therapy, and aide visits, agencies are expanding their scopes to provide services once available only in hospital settings.

The business of home health has also changed. In expanding to provide greater routine services, agencies rely on accounting systems and finance policies that allow for short- and long-term growth. These systems and policies help alleviate such "growing pains" as cash flow problems and finding adequate financing for expansion of plant and facilities.

In addition, voluntary agencies are applying for public and private grants to provide atypical services such as *Meals on Wheels* and *personal emergency response systems* that may not be covered by any third-party payer. Proprietary and voluntary home health organizations are adding additional sites and/or acquiring other organizations in a merger mania furor, as has occurred in other industries. In order to work well, these types of activities require specialized and innovative financing knowledge.

Given past changes, and being assured future changes will occur, it is important to be familiar with home health finance. This chapter will provide an introduction of the subject. Subsequent chapters will provide detail regarding accounting, finance, and third-party reimbursement.

# ACCOUNTING

Accounting is simply an information system for communicating financial facts and data. An accurate accounting system is necessary as a method of recording information that can be used to communicate meaningful data to interested parties. Financial data recorded during the agency's practice of business must be summarized in the form of financial statements, third-party reports, and other required schedules so that executives and administrators can make informed decisions. In today's home health environment, timely and accurate quantitative information is crucial in the decision-making process.

Agency management relies on accounting systems to provide information to answer basic operating questions. For instance:

QUESTION: Did the agency operate at a profit or loss for the current period?

ANSWER: *Profit/loss* (P/L), or *income statement*, reports summarize revenue and expense for a given period of time, such as a month, quarter, or year. This report can provide an immediate analysis of fiscal health and the earning potential of the agency.

QUESTION: What was the expense applicable to providing services to customers or patients?

ANSWER: The *Trial balance of expense*, or *cost report*, will report the direct expense for services provided and include applicable overhead. Overhead is the classification of expense not specifically associated with the production of identifiable products and services. Examples of such expense are utilities, depreciation, payroll taxes, and other administrative items. The cost report will allocate overhead to direct expense for purposes of calculating a cost per service or unit.

QUESTION: Are certain services or departments more efficient or profitable than others?

ANSWER: Financial analysis generated from an accounting system will enable management to determine whether one professional service or a particular department is more efficient than another. Also, it will help identify which class of payer is more profitable. Such information can be used as a guide in strategic management planning.

QUESTION: What is the agency's overall financial situation at a particular point in time?

ANSWER: The *Balance Sheet* statement summarizes the agency's assets, liabilities, and equity on a given date. Certain items, such as outstanding accounts receivable and loans due in the short term, highlight fiscal status.

QUESTION: How did the agency perform in relationship to its budget?

ANSWER: Monthly, quarterly, and annual financial reports should detail actual versus budgeted data to identify variances. These variances need to be questioned and adjustments made as needed.

QUESTION: Can financial and relevant statistical information be made available for internal and external reports?

ANSWER: *Internal Indicator reports* detailing utilization, revenue, and expense are helpful for agency management at all levels. *External Indicator reports* such as census, revenue and expense, and tax returns are required by various government, third-party insurance, and oversight organizations.

## Financial and Managerial Accounting

Financial accounting is confined to general purpose reports or financial statements directed to external users. External users have a primary interest in the review and evaluation of the operation and the financial status of the agency as a whole. Managerial accounting applies to internal reporting of financial data. Detailed information useful for management decision-making is obtained through managerial accounting reports.

# FINANCE

Today's businesses, including HHAs, face both short- and long-term financial concerns. An agency must have a clear financial vision as part of its overall strategic plan. Adequate cash reserves must be on hand to meet payrolls, applicable taxes, vendor bills, and other types of demand expenses. Financing must be secured for long-term capital expenditures such as new plant facilities, computer information systems, or capital improvements.

Finance is the proper management of money. *Revenue forecasts* are prepared to determine the profitability of the agency in the future. After visits are made and the revenue is recorded, the *accounts receivable* must be monitored and worked to bring the cash into the agency; uncollectible accounts must be written off. Cash flow analyses are needed to ensure current expenses are paid in a timely fashion.

## The Financial Manager

The role and responsibilities assigned to the manager of finance have expanded in recent times for three reasons.

- First, current economic times have seen mercurial inflation and interest rates. Management of funds invested and loans incurred requires obtaining the best possible rate and assuring the value of financial reserves do not deteriorate.
- Second, the complex and ever-changing environment of third-party reimbursement requires monitoring by the financial manager. Third-party receivables due from payers, or liabilities to be paid to payers, must be supervised for cash flow purposes. For instance, an agency may provide services in excess of its current reimbursement for a particular payer. The agency may now experience a cash flow problem since it has incurred the expense for these excess services, but is awaiting final payment (receivable) from the payer. Conversely, when the agency receives excess reimbursement for services provided, the agency will have to make a payment (liability) to the third-party payer. These financial situations require attentive cash flow planning and management.
- Third, agencies require long-term strategic financial plans to remain viable. If a new facility is required for expansion of services, then a thorough analysis is required to determine the future revenue and expenses applicable to the facility. This analysis will determine if a new facility is feasible in the near future, and what expenses will be incurred. Obtaining a precise analysis is difficult given fluctuating economic and reimbursement conditions. To allow for these conditions, a contingency budget may be developed.

# THIRD-PARTY REIMBURSEMENT

The fundamentals of accounting and finance are taught in business schools and applied to the basic operations of an agency. Previous accounting and finance experiences can be applied from other industries to the health care field. However, home health third-party reimbursement has nuances and idiosyncrasies that are best understood through experience within the field.

Home health third-party reimbursement is the reimbursement of expenses applicable to the provision of services to beneficiaries (patients). The primary third-party payers are Medicare (M/C), Medicaid (M/A), and commercial insurers such as Blue Cross. Each of the payers have unique reimbursement methodologies.

Unlike the prospective payment system of diagnostic related groupings (DRGs), M/C reimburses home health services under a retrospective, cost-based system.

Therefore the actual cost of providing services to M/C beneficiaries is the agency's reimbursement. The reimbursement rate is adjusted annually by the Health Care Financing Administration (HCFA) through its designated fiscal intermediaries (FI). This reimbursement is subject to routine cost limitations (cost limits, or caps) and other provisions.

Each state receives federal dollars to pay for health care provided to the indigent population. Medicaid administration reimbursement methodologies vary from state to state just as commercial insurers vary from plan to plan. Certain payers may utilize retrospective reimbursement, or they may utilize a prospective payment system (PPS), which involves determining a base year for costs and rolling those costs forward to a current year. Other payers may just establish a payment rate for a particular service and update it on an annual basis.

Reimbursement methodologies may vary or overlap among payers. It is important for financial management to understand the rules and methodologies to ensure adequate reimbursement for patient services provided. Individual state and third-party payer requirements will specify necessary reports to be filed, types of audits and reviews that will take place, and other protocols to be followed to avoid penalties or disallowances.

Medicare, as a payer, will be the focus of third-party reimbursement. Because M/C is the federal form of home health insurance, many other payers follow M/C in administering their reimbursement policies. Once versed in M/C regulations, it is easier to comprehend and work with other third-party reimbursement methodologies.

# FINANCIAL TABLE OF ORGANIZATION

Establishing an appropriate table of organization (T.O.) for an agency's financial department is the first step toward fiscal soundness. Identifying financial areas of responsibility and determining proper lines of reporting are crucial. Figure 9.1 is a sample of a functional financial table of organization.

Tables of organization vary depending on agency size, reporting responsibilities, and whether an agency is freestanding or hospital-based. Small agencies may have a simple T.O. with individuals or departments handling multiple tasks. In larger agencies the opposite is usually the case. Strategic planning may dictate how the T.O. of the finance department is structured.

Freestanding agencies may have a number of mid-level financial managers reporting to the chief financial officer (CFO), who then reports to the executive director. Hospital-based agencies might have a similar T.O. with a dotted line responsibility from the agency CFO to the finance department of the hospital. Figure 9.2 is an example of a large hospital-based financial T.O.

## Definition of Job Titles

Definitions of terms that identify job descriptions and functions of finance personnel in a typical freestanding agency might be helpful.

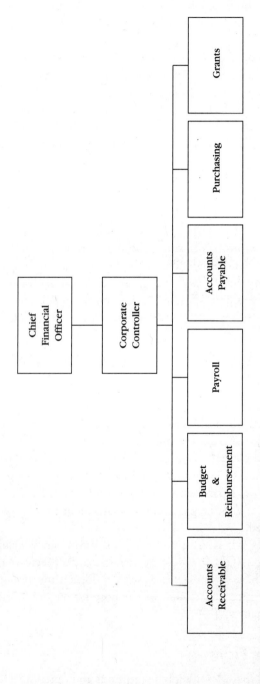

**FIGURE 9.1**  Functional Financial Table of Organization

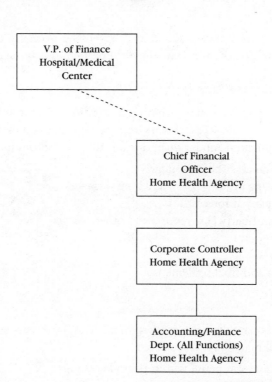

**FIGURE 9.2**   Hospital Based Home Health Agency Functional Table of Organization

## Chief Financial Officer

The CFO has overall responsibility for the accounting, finance, and reimbursement functions of an agency. Similar titles may be Vice President of Finance in a larger agency or Director of Finance in a smaller agency. Included in these responsibilities are financial statements, treasury management, accounts receivable/payable, annual budget, third-party reimbursement, and grants/special funds. The CFO may have responsibilities other than finance, such as administrative, support, and information system service functions.

## Corporate Controller

This position reports to the CFO and is responsible for the day-to-day financial operations of the agency. These responsibilities include preparation of cash flow analyses, payroll, petty cash, accounts payable, and grant/special fund requests. Also, the controller prepares interim and annual financial statements, which include the certification process by the outside independent auditors (to be discussed later in this chapter).

## Accounts Receivable (A/R) Manager

Primary responsibilities of this manager include timely third-party billing, assurance that collection procedures are adhered to, and the proper collection and deposit of cash receipts. An effective A/R manager is crucial, given the necessity of bringing in cash receipts at a rate that can accommodate the disbursement of payroll and other expenses.

### Budget/Reimbursement Manager

As the title indicates, this manager has responsibility over two different areas. However, both areas are related in scope of work and are dependent on each other. Most agencies combine both functions under one position. Responsibilities include

- preparation of annual corporate budget
- monthly monitoring of budget versus actual variances
- preparation of financial forecasts
- preparation of third-party cost reports and other filings
- third-party rate reviews
- third-party audits
- review of interim and final settlements.

### Payroll Manager

For most agencies payroll is the most significant expense associated with providing services. The payroll manager is responsible for

- proper classification of expense within payroll accounts
- disbursement of checks to employees
- payment of payroll taxes
- proper accounting of any company/employee deductions
- filing of local, state, and federal income tax forms and statements including W-2s.

### Accounts Payable (A/P) Manager

Disbursement of expense other than payroll is handled by the A/P manager who assures all administratively approved expense is disbursed to the appropriate vendors. Also, the A/P manager may set payment terms for vendors, such as terms that payment occurs sixty days after the service or invoice date.

### Purchasing Manager

The purchasing manager's responsibilities fall within two areas—materials management and finance. Procurement of clinical supplies, administrative stock, and minor equipment is the materials management component of this position. Arrangement for payment and the proper reporting of expense is the financial component. As a result of the financial component, the purchasing manager is usually included in the finance T.O.

### Grants Accountant

Certain agency activities not within the routine scope of visit services receive their financing in the form of grants. Grant monies, both revenue and expense, are kept separate from routine financial activities. It is the responsibility of the grants accountant to manage the recording of revenue and expense, and to complete necessary reporting requirements for interested parties.

## OUTSIDE INDEPENDENT AUDITORS

An agency prepares year-end financial statements to summarize annual operating results as well as to provide cost and statistical data for third-party reimbursement purposes. To assure accuracy of information, and as a requirement of third-party payers, agencies have outside independent auditors or certified public accountants (CPAs) express opinions on their financial statements.

The relationship between an agency and a CPA begins with the solicitation for a CPA to affirm, or *attest to,* the accuracy of the financial statements. After determining the scope of work required, the CPA firm will provide an engagement letter identifying the auditing services necessary and the fees for such services.

The audit involves a review of the financial record-keeping systems and verification of financial transactions utilizing statistical sampling methodologies. For HHAs, the scope of the audit will include a systems review of the process for the recording of visits and hours and how they are reported. As will be discussed in later chapters, these statistics are a major factor in determining revenue and expense.

The CPA will review and document such systems to gain an understanding of how the agency recognizes revenue and expense, and how service visits and hours are recorded. The CPA will then attest that the systems are functioning properly and have no material flaws. Last, they will determine if the A/R and agency investments are fairly presented.

To maintain a standard of consistency, those in the accounting profession have established rules and guidelines for auditing. In adhering to these practices, the agency management and outside interests are able to rely on the certified statements. A CPA may be held legally liable for any misrepresentations causing the user of the statements financial harm.

Audit findings that reveal errors or differences in financial valuations are discussed with agency management. Based on these discussions the general ledger is adjusted as necessary. Financial statements, with the auditor's opinion of fairness, are the final product.

The agency may utilize the CPA firm for services other than auditing, such as consulting services, installation of computerized accounting or data systems, tax work, or special assignments. Agencies may also call on CPA experience to evaluate the financial and legal aspects of any current problems or new ventures to be undertaken.

## CONCLUSION

In today's health care environment, the operation and management of an HHA requires the practice of sound financial fundamentals. Every aspect from cash flow to strategic financial budgeting is important for an agency's short- and long-term financial future.

The financial departments must be properly structured to operate efficiently and to anticipate the monetary concerns of the agency. Such departments will also provide relevant reports and information of value to all managerial levels.

## *Suggested Readings*

Brigham, E. F. & Gapenski, L. C. (1991). *Financial management: theory and practice.* Fort Worth, TX: The Dryden Press.

Garrison, R. H. (1991). *Managerial accounting—Concepts for planning, control, decision making.* Homewood, IL: Irwin.

Horngren, C. T. & Harrison, W. T. Jr. (1992). *Accounting.* Englewood Cliffs, NJ: Prentice Hall.

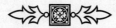

# CHAPTER

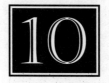

# Financial Statements and Definitions

**Timothy Riordan**

As mentioned in Chapter 9, an agency's accounting system provides financial data in the form of interim and annual reports. The reports that receive the most attention are the year-end, or certified, financial statements. These statements, or *financials,* contain

- reports of independent auditors
- balance sheet
- statement of revenue and expense
- statement of changes in financial position
- notes to financial statements

Once certified by the outside independent auditors, the financials provide indicators of past agency operating performance and current fiscal health. The financials are also utilized to prepare third-party cost reports and other required data schedules to determine reimbursement for services provided.

# REPORT OF INDEPENDENT AUDITORS

The auditor's report provides an opinion on the fairness of the statements, reports, supporting schedules, and notes contained within the agency's financials. The report is addressed to the governing body or others who have ultimate responsibility for the operation of the agency. It is this opinion that outside parties, such as third-party payers or organization investors, rely on to determine the fiscal status of the agency.

The standard auditor's report opens with the actual statements covered by his or her review for a defined period. This is followed by a disclosure informing readers that the financials are the responsibility of the organization's management, and that the auditor's primary function is to express an opinion on the fairness of the financials.

These statements are then followed by the *scope paragraph.* The scope paragraph identifies the financial and statistical reports and schedules covered by the opinion. It affirms that auditing standards and practices that are generally accepted by the accounting profession have been adhered to unless otherwise noted and described. Occasionally references are made if financial statements are examined by other auditors, particularly if data from prior periods have been used.

Auditor reports conclude with an *opinion paragraph.* Their opinion may be unqualified, or qualified. The majority of opinions are unqualified, or clean, meaning the financials are presented fairly in conformance with *generally accepted accounting principles* (GAAPs) that are consistently applied. Generally accepted accounting principles are guidelines of relatively detailed practices currently in use or adhered to in the accounting profession.

Material uncertainties in the statements or statistical reports result in qualifications. An example of a qualification is a discrepancy in valuing assets or other financial items. For instance, an agency may value its accounts receivable (A/R) at $2 million. A review by the auditor finds the A/R to be $1.5 million. If an understanding or adjustment cannot be agreed to, the auditor will render a qualified opinion to cover the discrepancy.

The following is an example of a Report of Independent Auditors that is dated on the last day of the field audit. It is addressed to the Board of Trustees of the agency for which it was prepared. The text is as follows:

We have audited the accompanying balance sheets of XYZ Home Health Agency (the Agency) as of December 31, 1994 and 1993, and the related statements of revenue and expense and changes in financial position for the years then ended. These financial statements are the responsibility of the Agency's management. Our responsibility is to express an opinion on these financial statements based on our audits.

We conducted our audits in accordance with generally accepted auditing standards. Those standards require that we plan and perform the audit to obtain reasonable assurance about whether the financial statements are free of material misstatement. An audit includes examining, on a test basis, evidence supporting the amounts and disclosures in the financial statements. An audit also includes assessing the accounting principles used and estimates made by management, as well as evaluating the overall financial statement presentation. We believe that our audits provide a reasonable basis for our opinion.

In our opinion, the financial statements referred to above present fairly, in all material respects, the financial position of the Agency at December 31, 1994 and 1993, and the results of its operations, changes in financial position for the years then ended in conformity with generally accepted accounting principles.

# BALANCE SHEET

The balance sheet presents the financial position of an agency at a specific date and reports *assets, liabilities, owner's equity,* and the relationship among them.

## Assets

Assets are the financial or economic resources that are recognized and measured in conformity with GAAP. They are classified into several types.

### Current Assets

Cash and cash equivalents, receivables for patient care, short-term investments, marketable securities, and inventories comprise current assets.

### Restricted Assets

Cash, cash equivalents, or other types of funds that are limited to a special purpose are considered restricted assets. The limitations are usually designated by the Board of Directors or, in the case of donated monies, in accordance with the donors' wishes.

### Long-Term Assets

Property, plant, equipment, and investments owned for a period of more than a year are included in this category.

## Liabilities

The opposite of assets are liabilities, which are financial or economic obligations that are recognized and measured in conformity with GAAP. They may be classified into *current liabilities* and *long-term liabilities*.

### Current Liabilities

Accounts payable and the current portion of long-term debt make up current liabilities. The current portion of long-term debt is the current year's obligation to service (pay) the debt. Also included are accrued liabilities, which are expenses that have actually been incurred, with payment expected to be made within twelve months.

### Long-Term Liabilities

Obligations that will not require the use of current assets within a time period of one year are considered long-term liabilities. Examples include long-term debt in the form of bonds and mortgages, or commitments incurred for construction of plant and facilities.

## Owner's Equity

The last component of the balance sheet is owner's equity, or what is more commonly referred to in the health care field as *fund balance*. The fund balance is the residual interest in assets after liabilities have been deducted. This amount is directly dependent upon agency management and the outside independent auditor's valuation of assets and liabilities.

Maintaining a positive fund balance is an indicator of good financial health and helps to assure the agency will be able to continue providing services in subsequent periods. Negative fund balances, on the other hand, raise doubts about an agency's survival, and cause concern among third-party payers and other oversight groups involved with the agency.

## STATEMENT OF REVENUE AND EXPENSE

The revenue and expense for services provided is recorded in the *general ledger* (GL) of the accounting system. The GL records all financial activities by classification of revenue and expense accounts. At the close of a particular time period, the GL is utilized to prepare the statement of revenue and expense, or as it is commonly known, the *profit/loss statement* (P/L).

Under GAAP, the accepted methodology of recording revenue and expense is the *accrual basis* of accounting. The accrual basis recognizes revenue when it is realized and expenses when incurred, regardless of the time of cash receipt or payment. This is important since revenue and expense will be matched with the actual visit service activity that occurred during the accounting time period.

The P/L is the report most often used by management to review financial performance. In part this is due to the frequency with which it is generated, usually on a monthly basis. A current P/L enables short-term planning and allows for timely corrections when necessary.

## Revenue Realization

The first step in determining revenue is to report all visit service utilization by discipline and payer generated by the management information system (MIS) of the agency. Paraprofessional services, in addition to being reported in visits, also require the reporting of hours in connection with those visits. This is due to the reimbursement of such services on an hourly basis by certain payers.

Once utilization is determined, the published charge for each service will be calculated to report *gross revenue*. Published charges are determined by the cost of each service. A charge is then published that is equal to or greater than the cost. The importance of published charges in third-party reimbursement will be discussed later.

Reimbursement rates, or the amount of payment per unit of service, promulgated by third-party payers are similarly assigned for each visit or hour of service to determine *net revenue.*. The difference between gross and net revenue is referred to as *contractual allowance*.

Once net revenue is determined, provisions should be made for insurer denials known as *bad debt*. Percentages are determined by evaluating current experience with billing and receipt of payment from various payers.

### *Patient Financial Assessment*

An important function in the accurate reporting and classification of revenue is to perform a *patient financial assessment* at the point of intake. The assessment should determine the patient's ability to pay, or what insurance will cover home care services provided.

The assessment for patients with Medicare (M/C) or Medicaid (M/A) coverage is fairly simple. Commercial insurance usually requires the agency to verify coverage with the patient's insurer.

The most difficult assessment is for private pay patients. These patients pay for services themselves as they do not have insurance coverage for home care services. In conducting the assessment, it may be noted that the private pay patient cannot afford the services charged.

At this point the agency may do one of three things. First, it may determine, in accordance with federal poverty guidelines, that the patient qualifies as charity care, in which case no payment is expected. Second, a sliding fee scale may be imposed whereby the patient pays only a percentage of the published charge. Last, a payment plan may be set up where periodic or installment payments are made by the patient.

# Expenses

An expense, or a cost, is the acquisition price of goods or services used in providing visits. Expenses for financial statements or cost reports are usually classified as *salaries, fringe benefits, contract services,* and *other.*

## Salaries

Payments made to agency employees at regular intervals for services rendered are considered salary. To earn the agreed-upon salary, the employee must work specified hours and perform the duties expected by the employer.

Agencies may augment a salary when the employee performs in an extraordinary manner. Additional amounts may be overtime (when an employee works more hours than required), bonuses (a reward for a positive result), or fee-for-service (a set dollar amount for visits or other services performed beyond the expected volume or panel of patients).

## Fringe Benefits

Benefits are expenses incurred and paid for by the employer to, or on behalf of, the employee in connection with wages and salaries. This is a separate expense over and above the employee's salary. Included in fringe benefits are the employee's portion of federal social security taxes, health insurance, pension plan, savings plan, and so forth.

## Contract Services

Money paid for services rendered by parties outside the agency, either individuals or organizations, are contract expenses. Examples of services provided under contract are clinical (nursing, physical, occupational, or speech therapy, medical social work, or home health aide), management (accounting or consulting), clerical (mail room out sourcing), and maintenance (cleaning).

## Other Expenses

Other types of expenses an agency may incur are depreciation of plant and equipment, rent, legal, clinical, office supplies, and utilities, among others. Standard financial reporting have these expenses reported in separate accounts on the GL.

## Direct and Overhead Expenses

Expenses may also be categorized as *direct* or *overhead.* Direct expenses are incurred with the actual, or hands-on, provision of clinical services. Nursing salaries, medical supplies, and contracted home health aide services are all examples of direct expense. Overhead expenses are incurred for the administrative support of clinical services. Examples include supervision, case management, accounting, and billing for visits.

The categorization of direct and overhead expenses can be confusing when dealing with the costs of an agency that has a sponsoring organization. The sponsoring organization considers the entire agency cost, both direct and overhead, as direct. Such is the case with a hospital-based agency where the agency administrator's salary is considered direct expense by the sponsoring organization, although the position does not provide clinical services to patients.

### Cost Account or Center

It is important for expenses that are similar in nature to be grouped and reported in their proper *cost account* or *cost center*. The general ledger has a *chart of accounts* listing all cost accounts and centers available for reporting expense.

For example, if an agency has direct-care nurses and physical therapists, then salaries for each group should be reported in separate accounts. Expenses other than salary should also be treated in a similar fashion. Expenses applicable to a building would be reported in a maintenance cost account separate from other cost accounts.

## STATEMENT OF CHANGES IN FINANCIAL POSITION (EQUITY)

A statement of changes in financial position is a requirement for certified financial statements. This statement summarizes the financing and investment activities of the agency, including the extent to which the agency has generated funds from operations during the year. The basic purpose of the statement is to disclose the activities of working capital or monetary funds of the agency.

The statement also discloses significant changes even if they do not affect working capital.

For instance, a publicly owned home care company may issue a note or security to obtain property. Even though the company's working capital is not affected, the proceeds of the issuance is a source of funds and the property is a use of funds.

## NOTES TO THE FINANCIAL STATEMENTS

Certain information about an agency's financial position may not be apparent from reading the financial statements. To provide adequate disclosure, it is usually necessary to supplement the financial statements with additional information in the form of notes to the financial statements.

The notes usually include a description of the organization and a summary of significant accounting policies utilized to prepare the statements. Third-party reimbursement programs, summary of property, plant and equipment, leases, long-term debt, and pension plans are described in the notes. If agencies are facing legal claims or other uncertainties, these contingencies are reported in financial notes, as well.

# THE "BOTTOM LINE"

The question "what is the bottom line?" has different meanings for different situations, such as for freestanding versus hospital-based agencies. The profitability of an agency is noted on the P/L (the surplus of revenue over expense or the deficit of expense over revenue). One should not just consider revenue minus expense, but *extraordinary* revenue and expense items as well.

### Case Study

ABC Agency has a current period loss of $500,000—$12 million in revenue and $12.5 million in expense. The loss gives the appearance of nonprofitability or inefficiency. However, the agency had an organizational restructuring that resulted in a one-time charge of $700,000 against earnings. Therefore instead of a $500,000 loss, the real profit from operations is $200,000.

This charge should be separately reported on the P/L statement as an extraordinary item and also documented in the notes. Such reporting would give the reader a more accurate number on the profitability from operations, or the real bottom line.

In addition to extraordinary items, hospital-based agencies require special attention to overhead expense allocated from the sponsoring organization. A hospital-based agency will have its own direct expense from patient care, and its own overhead from agency administrative support services. The agency incurs additional overhead expense from the hospital for services such as payroll, employee health, legal services, and so forth.

In presenting a P/L statement, it is important to identify the hospital-allocated overhead. Reporting it as a separate expense item will help senior hospital management determine the profitability of the agency. Profitability, or the bottom line, is *contribution to overhead.*

# CONCLUSION

Reviewing financial statements provides a measure of understanding of a home health agency's fiscal health. Both internal agency management and interested third-party payers and regulators read and use financial statements.

The balance sheet provides an indicator of long-term viability of the agency, whereas the P/L reports current fiscal affairs. Certification of the financial statements by independent auditors provides increased reliability of the reporting, thereby giving readers and users additional assurance or confidence.

## *Suggested Readings*

Brigham, E. F. & Gapenski, L. C. (1991). *Financial management: Theory and practice.* Fort Worth, TX: The Dryden Press.

Horngren, C. T. and Harrison, W. T. Jr. (1992). *Accounting.* Englewood Cliffs, NJ: Prentice Hall.

# CHAPTER

# 11

# Medicare Reimbursement Principles

**Timothy Riordan**

Home health third-party reimbursement mechanisms vary from payer to payer. Some use a cost-based (retrospective) methodology; others use a prospective payment system, or, as commercial insurers do, utilize a fee for service schedule.

Regardless of the form of reimbursement, each is a derivative of the federal payer of home health services, Medicare (M/C). Since M/C beneficiaries are found throughout the country, individual state Medicaid (M/A) plans and regional commercial insurers are well aware of M/C reimbursement principles; thus, they model reimbursement after M/C. Payer philosophy and budgetary concerns affect reimbursement principles, which in turn affect the coverage of services.

This chapter will describe primary M/C reimbursement principles utilized by the *Health Care Financing Administration* (HCFA) in determining payment for home health services. It should be noted that these principles are applied by the *fiscal intermediaries* (FI) across the country. Therefore certain principles may be subject to slightly different interpretations, depending on the geographical region.

Complicating the situation is the further subdivision by HCFA into ten regions of FI services. Each regional area has a designated FI to process M/C claims submitted by all types of agencies; these FIs are known as *regional home health intermediaries* (RHHIs). The RHHI is responsible for the cost reporting and rate setting processes for *freestanding* agencies. The cost reporting and rate setting processes for *hospital-based* agencies is handled by the FI in charge of the sponsoring hospital. Therefore within the same geographic region, M/C principles may be subject to different interpretation. Additionally, for a hospital-based agency the FI and RHHI may be in two separate areas of the country, as is the case in New York State where the FI is in Region II and the RHHI is in Region V.

# MEDICARE REIMBURSEMENT OF PROPER AND REASONABLE COST

The current M/C methodology of reimbursement for home health services is *cost-based*, or *retrospective*. All costs applicable to agency operations are reported on a *cost report*. These costs are then subjected to an allocation and apportionment process to determine M/C reimbursable cost. Discussion of the cost report process will follow in Chapter 12.

The first principle governing M/C home health reimbursement is that the costs associated with providing care to beneficiaries are *proper* and *reasonable*. This principle is applied to both direct and indirect (overhead) costs associated with the provision of home health service(s).

Proper and reasonable costs are required for all patients irrespective of payment source. This is to ensure that in the apportionment process, final M/C reimbursement does not include excess costs pertaining to other payers, and conversely other payers do not reimburse for excess M/C cost.

In determining if costs are proper and reasonable, the FI takes into account the prevailing costs of providing services within the agency's geographic area. Any cost that appears to be outside the prevailing geographic cost will be examined by the FI. If the expense is excessive, the FI will adjust the expense down to a level determined to be proper and reasonable.

There are justifiable instances when an agency may incur excess costs due to situations beyond its control.

For example, an agency may have problems receiving home medical equipment (HME) from a local area vendor due to poor product quality or delivery service. The agency contracts with a higher quality and more reliable vendor outside its area. Excess costs are incurred due to better products and the distance involved with delivery. When queried by the FI, explanation and documentation should result in no disallowance being made.

# COSTS RELATED TO PATIENT CARE

The recording of costs is as important to home health agencies (HHAs) as it is to any other business. However, the reporting of costs for M/C purposes is subject to special provisions usually not applicable to other businesses.

## Adequate Cost Data and Cost Finding

*Adequate cost data* and *cost finding* are mandated by HCFA in order to develop the reimbursement rate for M/C beneficiaries served by an agency. Adequate cost data is substantiated by a provider maintaining supporting documentation for all expenses reported on the cost report. Such documentation includes general ledgers, receipts, and any pertinent accounting/financial schedules or analysis. This documentation will be reviewed by the FI when the audit of the cost report is performed.

Cost finding means that statistical allocations and other methodologies utilized on the cost report are in accordance with M/C regulations and generally accepted accounting principles; these too are subject to audit.

## Prudent Buyer Principle

Incurring costs for goods and services requires agency management to observe the *prudent buyer* principle. This principle requires the agency to obtain the best price for a good or service without compromising the quality of patient care. Examples of prudent buyer include volume discounts on contract home health aide hourly purchases or obtaining bids from different suppliers to determine the best price for paper, pens, and other office supplies.

Every agency should have a written policy and procedure regarding purchasing. The procedure should require a minimum of three bids from different vendors for the purchase of goods and services over a specified dollar amount. Presentation to the FI of the written policy/procedure, and evidence it is followed, will support that the agency's costs are reasonable and not excessive.

## Liquidation of Liabilities

The accrual basis of accounting requires the recording of expense at the actual time it is incurred, no matter when payment is made. This results in the expense being reported in the cost report for the appropriate time period. Until the actual payment is made, the agency records the expense as a liability on the balance sheet.

To properly record M/C reimbursement of paid expense, HCFA instituted the *liquidation of liability* principle. Within one year, after the end of the cost reporting period, short-term expense must be paid, thereby eliminating the liability from the balance sheet. If a liability is not liquidated, or paid, within the required time frame, the FI will not allow the expense to be included in the cost report. The expense may be included in a subsequent cost report if the liability is liquidated during that time period.

### Case Study

An agency engages a consultant to perform a research project. The agency accrues the consultant expense at the time the contract goes into effect, although the fees will not be paid until the research is completed. However, during the contract life there is a dispute and the research is never finished. The agency refuses to pay any fee, but does not reverse the accrual entry of expense.

On audit, the FI reviews consulting expense and disallows the expense because it was not paid during the cost report year. If the dispute is resolved in a subsequent time period and payment is made, the FI will allow for reimbursement of expense.

# TREATMENT OF SPECIFIC COSTS

Certain expenses reported on the cost report require mentioning since they are almost always reviewed by the FI. These expenses are *depreciation, interest,* and *owner's compensation.*

## Depreciation

An agency that purchases buildings or equipment, or makes other significant capital acquisitions, charges the cost to the appropriate balance sheet asset accounts. Although these assets may provide services for a number of years, eventually they will have to be replaced. Therefore, the cost of each asset must be spread over its estimated useful life. This is depletion or depreciation of the asset, and the associated cost reported in each year is known as depreciation expense.

Medicare regulations allow for the reimbursement of depreciation applicable to agency assets; they specify the allowable depreciation calculation methodologies. *Straight-line, declining balance* and *sum of years' digits* will be discussed.

### Straight Line

The most common manner of calculating depreciation expense is the straight-line method. Using this method the cost of the asset is distributed evenly over the life of the asset.

For example, an agency purchases a $3,000,000 facility that is expected to provide operating space for 30 years. The depreciation expense per year using the straight-line method is $100,000 ($3,000,000 divided by 30 years).

### Declining Balance and Sum of the Years' Digits

Other more complicated depreciation methods, declining balance and sum of the years' digits, are used by agencies to accelerate the reporting of depreciation expense. This has the effect of "speeding up" the reimbursement of expense applicable to the asset.

The FI will review *plant ledgers* detailing the purchase price of assets and depreciation expense recorded. The review will encompass the cost of the asset, the life of the asset, salvage values, and depreciation methodologies.

## Interest

Agencies normally have to borrow money to help ease situations of tight cash flow or to finance major purchases and expansion. The cost applicable to such borrowing is termed interest expense. Medicare reimburses for interest expense that is proper, reasonable, and required for the provision of agency services to beneficiaries.

The FI reviews interest expense loan agreements to

1. ensure monies were borrowed
2. ensure the interest rate is reasonable
3. require payment of interest and repayment of the funds.

If the FI's review shows borrowing was not necessary, or the interest rate was usurious or unreasonable, a partial or total disallowance of interest payments will occur.

## Owner's Compensation

Proprietary HHAs that compensate the owner, owners, or owner's relatives for services rendered will have the arrangement reviewed by the FI. The review of owner's compensation is conducted to ensure the cost for such services is necessary and reasonable.

Necessary means the services of the owner are required for agency operations and that the agency would have to make arrangements to have the services provided by someone else if not attended to by the owner. Reasonableness requires the compensation paid for such services is not excessive compared to what is paid by other agencies in the same market.

The FI requires proprietary agencies to complete owner compensation questionnaires. These questionnaires request details on compensation packages of owners, their job descriptions and functions, owner academic and professional backgrounds, and the size of the agency.

Based on this questionnaire, the FI can determine the reasonableness of the compensation under review. Any compensation deemed excessive by the FI will be eliminated from reimbursable costs.

The FI may also request compensation scales of the chief executive officer (CEO) and other high-level management positions in voluntary agencies. Any determination of excessiveness in a compensation package may result in a disallowance.

The subject of owner's compensation is usually a sensitive matter. To prevent disallowances, agencies should properly document job descriptions and responsibilities. Salary and compensation packages of agency officers should have the approval of the Board of Directors. Last, the agency should be prepared to discuss with the FI the appropriateness of the compensation package.

# TREATMENT OF INCOME

The total operations of an HHA generate a number of income streams. These streams include *ordinary income, ancillary income, purchase discounts and allowances,* and *grant income.*

## Ordinary Income

The services provided by an agency are reimbursed by various third-party payers in accordance with their regulations. This revenue is considered ordinary patient service income and usually is not considered in the determination of M/C reimbursable cost.

## Ancillary Income

However, an agency may receive other forms of revenue that will be reviewed by the FI in determining reimbursable cost. Examples of such income are vending machine income, purchase discounts, and other nonpatient care revenue.

The theory behind the FI review is that expense may be incurred in the generation of nonpatient care revenue. This expense may be reported with other expenses incurred in the provision of patient care and thus be included in the calculation of M/C reimbursement. To prevent such a situation, either the expense must be identified and excluded, or the expense has to be reduced by the applicable revenue.

### Case Study

An agency has a candy vending machine on its property, and incurs expenses for the products sold and the utilities required to operate the machine. The expense associated with operating the machine is not considered to be patient care related, and therefore not reimbursable by M/C.

It is very difficult for the FI to identify the exact expense necessary to be excluded from M/C reimbursable expense. A reasonable solution to this is to offset the revenue from the vending machine against agency administrative cost. The methodology may not be exact, but it is close enough, and any difference of M/C reimbursement would be immaterial.

## Purchase Discounts and Allowances

The FI will also review purchase rebates and volume discounts received by the agency. These rebates and discounts are not revenue but actually a reduction of expense. Medicare reimbursable cost should be adjusted to account for such a reduction.

An example will be helpful. In vendor contracting for home health aide hourly services, an agency agrees to purchase at $12 per hour. The contract provides for a $1 per hour discount if 10,000 hours are purchased. The agency purchases 10,000 hours and records expense of $120,000 (10,000 hours multiplied by $12 per hour). This results in a purchase discount of $10,000 (10,000 hours multiplied by $1 per hour). Medicare reporting requires that the $120,000 expense be reduced by the $10,000 purchase discount to properly reflect the expense.

## Grant Income

Agencies may be requested to provide atypical services by not-for-profit entities or other philanthropic causes. These organizations agree to fund the expense of such services by providing grant monies to agencies. The agency reports these monies as *grant income.*

Income from grants also needs to be addressed for M/C reimbursable cost issues. Discussion of this topic will be addressed in Chapter 12, *Medicare Cost Reporting.*

# LOWER OF COST OR CHARGES

In determining final M/C reimbursement for patient care services, the FI performs a *lower of cost or charges* (LCC) comparison. The LCC provision compares the reimbursement of reasonable cost to the customary charges for those services. The lower of the two is considered final reimbursement for M/C services.

In the comparison, both cost and charges are compared in the aggregate as opposed to a per discipline or disaggregate basis. Therefore aggregation has the benefit of allowing charges to be lower than cost for one service but higher than cost in another. The excess cost over charges for a particular service is then offset by the lower-than-cost service.

## Principle of Lower of Cost or Charges

### Case Study

Patient A has M/C coverage and requires skilled nursing and physical therapy services while on home care. Patient B is private pay and receives the exact same services. The agency has a published charge schedule with an individual charge for each service. Under the M/C definition of "customary charges," the charges for each service are uniformly applied to all payers. Certain payers that have a fixed rate of payment under a contract with the agency are exempt from the uniformly applied condition.

In the example, the services rendered to both patients has resulted in charges of $100 per visit, or $1,000 for ten visits. Bills are sent to M/C for Patient A and to Patient B for himself.

Upon subsequent final settlement of the M/C cost report by the FI, a final cost per visit of $95 is calculated. As the charge of $100 per visit is greater than the cost of $95 per visit, the provider will receive full reimbursement of $95 per visit for all M/C services rendered.

If a cost per visit of $105 was calculated, the LCC provision would have final reimbursement at $100, the charge per visit. The provider would lose $5 per visit of M/C reimbursement.

The theory behind LCC for the disallowance is that M/C will not pay $5 more per visit than the private pay patient for the exact same services. Paying the additional $5 per visit has the effect of M/C subsidizing private pay patients.

Application of LCC requires an agency to know the *cost* for services, and then establish proper charges that will not result in the loss of M/C reimbursement. The process of establishing charges for agency services is similar to any nonhealth care business. Through the budget and cost accounting process, an agency should be able to determine the cost for individual services prior to the start of the fiscal year (FY).

From the individual *cost per unit*, the agency should establish an individual *charge per unit* that is equal to or greater than the cost per unit. An appropriate *safety margin* between cost and charge should be considered. If unpredicted additional expense is incurred by the agency during the FY, the safety margin will help ensure the higher-than-budgeted cost per visit is not jeopardized when the M/C cost report is filed.

It should be noted that charges are not set for any particular period of time, and can be revised whenever necessary. Periodic reviews of the relationship of cost to charges should be made during the FY.

Also, a consideration in the establishment of published charges are the charges of other agencies in the same locality. An agency with excessive charges may lose private pay business or be confronted by a community oversight group.

## Carryover of Nonreimbursed Costs

Prior to 1986, the LCC provision included a two-year carryover feature for reimbursement lost to LCC. If an agency was penalized for $30,000 in reimbursable cost in excess of charges, the agency has the subsequent two-year time period to adjust charges to be higher than costs. The amount of charges in excess of cost would be utilized to recover up to the $30,000 in lost reimbursement.

This provision was eliminated by HCFA in 1986 under the assumption an agency should be able to estimate its costs for the upcoming year and properly establish charges. Such logic requires an agency to accurately budget costs for an upcoming year, monitor these costs during the year, and adjust charges if necessary.

Government operated HHAs receive special considerations under LCC as a result of their *public status*. Charges can be 50 percent or less than cost and there will be no penalty imposed by M/C. The patient population of public providers are usually those who have little or no insurance coverage, or are indigent.

For a public agency to qualify for the LCC exemption, the agency must establish a *no-charge* or *nominal charge* structure. No-charge is simply not charging for services, and nominal charge is a charge that is at 50 percent or less of the cost of the services.

Adhering to these charge structures will result in full reimbursement of M/C cost. The importance of maintaining a nominal charge structure at 50 percent or less of cost cannot be overemphasized. Any percentage higher than 50 percent may result in the FI determining that the charge structure is not nominal. This may prove disastrous and could lead to a significant loss of M/C reimbursement.

## CONCLUSION

Familiarity with M/C reimbursement principles is essential for the fiscal health of an agency. Diligent financial management that assesses the implications of day-to-day transactions, and establishment and revision of published charges, will position the agency to make sound decisions.

The FI audit of a cost report is a traumatic experience for most agencies. Anxiety will be eased if the agency has the same level of expertise as the auditors.

## *Suggested Reading*

U.S. Department of Health and Human Services Health Care Financing Administration. 1994. *Medicare provider reimbursement manual HCFA–Pub. 15-1*. Chapters 1, 2, 8, 9, 21, 23, & 26.

# CHAPTER

## 12

# Medicare Cost Reporting

**Timothy Riordan**

Because Medicare (M/C) reimbursement for home health care is cost-based and retrospective, a document is required for agencies to report expenses. This document is the *cost report*.

The original home health agency (HHA) cost report (1966) consisted of two pages. Since then, the document has evolved into a complicated and sophisticated process, as has nearly everything else in the home care business.

Cost reports are different for freestanding and hospital-based agencies. Freestanding agencies utilize the *HCFA-1728* and, as discussed in Chapter 11, it is filed with their designated regional home health intermediary (RHHI) on an annual basis.

Hospital-based agencies report their information and costs with the sponsoring hospital's cost report. These agencies report on *Supplemental Worksheet H Schedules* of the *HCFA-2552*. This report ensures proper allocations of hospital expense to the agency. The entire hospital cost report is filed with the FI on an annual basis.

This chapter will detail the worksheets and schedules of the HCFA-1728, since it contains many similarities to the HCFA-2552. A section will be devoted to their differences, as well.

# HCFA-1728 WORKSHEETS

## Preliminary Schedules

The first HCFA-1728 schedules to be completed are *Worksheets S and S-1*. Worksheet S records general demographic information about the HHA filing the cost report. Included is agency name and address, six-digit provider number, and other data about the provider. Figure 12.1 is a reproduction of Worksheet S.

On the worksheet is a certification statement indicating that the cost and other information is complete and properly reported to the best knowledge and belief of the agency. The certification must be signed by an officer or director of the agency.

### Worksheet S-1

Worksheet S-1 has two sections, *statistical* and *employment data*. Statistical data requires information on visits and patients served per discipline, unduplicated census, and total home health aide hours rendered. The unduplicated census is the total number of patients seen during the reporting year. No patient is counted more than once, regardless of the number of times the patient may have been readmitted during the year. These statistics are to be reported in two categories, M/C, or Title XVIII, and all other payers.

Employment data requests full-time equivalents (FTEs) for both employees and contract services. The FTEs are to be reported in ten specific job titles. For S-1 purposes, the FTEs must be calculated utilizing an equivalency factor of: 2,080 hours per year equals one FTE.

The 2,080 hours per year equates to forty hours per week. This may cause FTE reporting problems for agencies who utilize anything less than a forty-hour work week. To resolve this problem, agencies should first determine paid hours for employees during the year. Then these paid hours can be divided by 2,080 to determine FTEs for S-1.

**Case Study**

An agency may have work hours of 8:30 A.M. to 5:00 P.M. daily, and 30 nurses are employed. Each nursing employee works 7.5 hours per day (allowing 1 hour off for lunch), 37.5 hours per week (7.5 hours per day multiplied by 5 days per week), and 1,950 hours per year (37.5 hours per week multiplied by 52 weeks per year).

Assuming only regular hours (no overtime) are worked for the entire year, total paid nursing hours are 58,500 (1,950 hours per employee multiplied by 30 employees). Nursing FTEs to be reported on S-1 are 28.13 (58,500 paid hours divided by 2,080 hours per FTE).

Figure 12.2 is a reproduction of Worksheet S-1.

## Classification of Expense

The first step in determining M/C reimbursement is to classify agency expense on the cost report. The accepted classification of expense is reported on

- *Worksheet A:* Reclassification and Adjustment of Trial Balance of Expense. Trial balance of expense is a list prepared at the end of a reporting period detailing expense account titles and balances.
- *Worksheet A-1:* Compensation Analysis Salaries and Wages
- *Worksheet A-2:* Compensation Analysis Employee Benefits
- *Worksheet A-3:* Compensation Analysis Contracted Services/Purchased Services

The titles of the Worksheets A through A-3 explain the types of expense to be reported in each one. Figures 12.3, 12.4, 12.5, and 12.6 are reproductions of Worksheets A through A-3.

Worksheet A can be considered a summary schedule because totals from A-1 through A-3 are transferred to it. In addition, Worksheet A provides for the reporting of expense that is not salaries, fringes, or contract services such as purchased home health aide hours. Other such expenses are reported in *column 5, other costs.*

Each worksheet is divided into columns and rows. At the top of each column is a title for a particular type of expense. Worksheets A-1 through A-3 have the following column titles for expense: administrators, directors, supervisors, nurses, therapists, aides, and all other.

In reporting expense on these schedules, the expense is classified by which column it belongs in. For example, physical therapist salaries would be reported on Worksheet A-1, *column 6, therapists.*

FORM APPROVED
OMB NO. 0938-0022

This report is required by law (42 USC 1395g; 42 CFR 413.20(b)). Failure to report can result in all interim payments made since the beginning of the cost reporting period being deemed overpayments (42 USC 1395g).

| HOME HEALTH AGENCY COST REPORT | | WORKSHEET S |
|---|---|---|
| Intermediary Use Only<br>[ ] Audited<br>[ ] Desk Reviewed | Intermediary Number | Date Received |

PART I—GENERAL

| 1 NAMES AND ADDRESSES | PROVIDER NUMBER | DATES CERTIFIED |
|---|---|---|
| HOME HEALTH AGENCY | | |
| HOME HEALTH BASED HOSPICE | | |
| HOME HEALTH BASED CORF | | |

2 AGENCY IDENTIFIER

1. [ ]   Combination Official and Voluntary

2. [ ]   Official

   a. [ ]  Federal   b. [ ]  State   c. [ ]  City

   d. [ ]  City - County   e. [ ]  County   f. [ ]  Health District

3. [ ]   Voluntary Non-Profit

   a. [ ]  Church   b. [ ]  Other Than Church

4. [ ]   Private—Non-profit

5. [ ]   Proprietary

   a. [ ]  Sole Proprietor   b. [ ]  Corp.   c. [ ]  Partnership

PART II—CERTIFICATION BY OFFICER OR DIRECTOR OF THE AGENCY

INTENTIONAL MISREPRESENTATION OR FALSIFICATION OF ANY INFORMATION CONTAINED
IN THIS COST REPORT MAY BE PUNISHABLE BY FINE AND/OR IMPRISONMENT UNDER FEDERAL LAW

I HEREBY CERTIFY that I have read the above statement and that I have examined the accompanying
Home Health Agency Cost Report and the Balance Sheet and the Statement of Revenue and Expenses
prepared by _____ and
(Provider name(s) and number(s) for the cost report beginning _____
ending _____, and that to the best of my knowledge and belief, it is
a true, correct and complete report prepared from the books and records of the provider in
accordance with applicable instructions, except as noted.


_____        _____        _____
(Signed)                                  Title                              Date
Officer or Director


Annual reporting burden and recordkeeping burden is estimated at 160 hours per recordkeeper. This includes time for reviewing

instructions, searching existing data sources, gathering and maintaining data needed, and completing and reviewing the collection of

information. Send comments regarding this burden estimate or any other aspects of this collection of information, including suggestions

for reducing the burden, to Health Care Financing Administration, P.O. Box 26684, Baltimore, Md. 21207, and to the Office of Information

and Regulatory Affairs, Office of Management and Budget, Washington, D.C. 20503. Paperwork Reduction Project (0938–0022).

FORM HCFA–1728-86 (Amended 12/92)(12/92) (INSTRUCTIONS FOR THIS WORKSHEET ARE PUBLISHED IN
    HCFA 15–II, SECTION 1701–1701.2)

**FIGURE 12.1**    Worksheet S

| HOME HEALTH AGENCY STATISTICAL DATA | PROVIDER NO.: _____ | PERIOD: FROM _____ TO _____ | WORKSHEET S-1 |

PART 1—STATISTICAL DATA

| | Title XVIII | | Other | | Total | |
|---|---|---|---|---|---|---|
| | Visits | Patients | Visits | Patients | Visits | Patients |
| | 1 | 2 | 3 | 4 | 5 | 6 |
| 1 Skilled Nursing | | | | | | |
| 2 Physical Therapy | | | | | | |
| 3 Speech Pathology | | | | | | |
| 4 Occupational Therapy | | | | | | |
| 5 Medical Social Service | | | | | | |
| 6 Home Health Aide | | | | | | |
| 7 All Other Services | | | | | | |
| 8 Total Visits | | | | | | |
| 9 Unduplicated Census Count | | | | | | |
| 10 Home Health Aide Hours | | | | | | |

144

PART II—EMPLOYMENT DATA

| Employment Category | Staff No. of FTE Employees (2080 hrs) | Contract No. of FTE Employees (2080 hrs) | Total |
|---|---|---|---|
| | 1 | 2 | 3 |
| 1 Nurses[1]—RNs | | | |
| 1a —LPN | | | |
| 1b —LVN | | | |
| 2 Physical Therapists | | | |
| 3 Speech Pathologists | | | |
| 4 Occupational Therapists | | | |
| 5 Medical Social Workers | | | |
| 6 Home Health Aides[2] | | | |
| 7 Executive Administrative Personnel[3] | | | |
| 8 Financial Administrative Personnel[4] | | | |
| 9 General Administrative Personnel[5] | | | |
| 10 Other[6] | | | |
| | | | |
| | | | |

[1] This category includes all nurses, i.e., RNs, LPNs, LVNs. A nurse supervisor (if part of her time is spent performing visits) should be included in this category.

[2] Includes homemakers.

[3] Includes administrators, assistant administrators, directors, assistant directors, and supervisors (if sole function is administrative).

[4] Includes accountants, internal auditors, statisticians and other professional financial personnel.

[5] Includes categories such as billing, payroll clerks, secretaries, telephone operators, personnel specialists, security personnel, maintenance staff, and other administrative employees.

[6] Any other employee classifications. These include, but are not limited to respiratory therapists, nutritionists, and any other employee not included in any of the other employee classifications.

FORM HCFA-1728-86 (INSTRUCTIONS FOR THIS WORKSHEET ARE PUBLISHED IN BCFA PUB. 15-11 SECS. 1702-702.2) (12-92)

**Figure 12.2**  Worksheet S-1

145

### RECLASSIFICATION AND ADJUSTMENT OF TRIAL BALANCE OF EXPENSES

| | | SALARIES (Fr Wks A-1) | EMPLOYEE BENEFITS (Fr Wks A-2) | TRANSPOR-TATION (See Instructions) | CONTRACTED PURCHASED SERVICES (Fr Wks A-3) |
|---|---|---|---|---|---|
| | | 1 | 2 | 3 | 4 |
| | **GENERAL SVC COST CTRS** | | | | |
| 1 | Cap Rel—Bldg & Fix | | | | |
| 2 | Cap Rel—Mov Equip | | | | |
| 3 | Plant Oper & Maint. | | | | |
| 4 | Transp. (See Instruc) | | | | |
| 5 | Admin. & General | | | | |
| | **HHA REIMBURSABLE SVCS** | | | | |
| 6 | Skilled Nursing Care | | | | |
| 7 | Physical Therapy | | | | |
| 8 | Occupational Therapy | | | | |
| 9 | Speech Pathology | | | | |
| 10 | Med Social Services | | | | |
| 11 | Home Health Aide | | | | |
| 12 | DME—Rented | | | | |
| 13 | DME—Sold | | | | |
| 14 | Supplies (See Instruc) | | | | |
| | **HHA NONREIMBURSABLE SERVICES** | | | | |
| 15 | Home Dialy. Aide Svcs | | | | |
| 16 | Respiratory Therapy | | | | |
| 17 | Private Duty Nursing | | | | |
| 18 | Clinic | | | | |
| 19 | Hlth Promotion Activ. | | | | |
| 20 | Day Care Program | | | | |
| 21 | Home Delivered Meals Program | | | | |
| 22 | CORF | | | | |
| | **SPECIAL PURPOSE COST CENTER** | | | | |
| 23 | Hospice | | | | |
| | **OTHER NONREIMBURSABLE COSTS** | | | | |
| 24 | Homemaker Service | | | | |
| 25 | Other | | | | |
| | **OTHER COSTS** | | | | |
| 26 | Insurance—Malpractice | | | | |
| 27 | Insurance—Other | | | | |
| 28 | Interest | | | | |
| 29 | TOTAL | | | | |

FORM HCFA-1728-86 (INSTRUCTIONS FOR THIS WORKSHEET ARE PUBLISHED IN HCFA PUB. 15-11, SEC. 1703) (12-92)

**FIGURE 12.3** Worksheet A

| | | PROVIDER NO.: | PERIOD: FROM ——————————— TO ——————————— | | WORKSHEET A |
|---|---|---|---|---|---|

| | OTHER COSTS | TOTAL AGENCY COST | RECLASSI-FICATION (Fr Wks A-4) | RECLASSI-FIED TRIAL BALANCE (Cols 6 ± 7) | ADJUSTMENTS TO EXPENSES (INCR/DECR) (Fr Wks A-5) | FOR COST ALLOCATION (Col 8 ± 9) | |
|---|---|---|---|---|---|---|---|
| | 5 | 6 | 7 | 8 | 9 | 10 | |
| | | | | | | | |
| | | | | | | | 1 |
| | | | | | | | 2 |
| | | | | | | | 3 |
| | | | | | | | 4 |
| | | | | | | | 5 |
| | | | | | | | 6 |
| | | | | | | | 7 |
| | | | | | | | 8 |
| | | | | | | | 9 |
| | | | | | | | 10 |
| | | | | | | | 11 |
| | | | | | | | 12 |
| | | | | | | | 13 |
| | | | | | | | 14 |
| | | | | | | | 15 |
| | | | | | | | 16 |
| | | | | | | | 17 |
| | | | | | | | 18 |
| | | | | | | | 19 |
| | | | | | | | 20 |
| | | | | | | | 21 |
| | | | | | | | 22 |
| | | | | | | | 23 |
| | | | | | | | 24 |
| | | | | | | | 25 |
| | | | ( ) | -0- | | | 26 |
| | | | ( ) | -0- | | | 27 |
| | | | ( ) | -0- | | | 28 |
| | | | -0- | | | | 29 |

COMPENSATION ANALYSIS
SALARIES AND WAGES

| | ADMINIS-TRATORS | DIRECTORS | CONSULTANTS | |
|---|---|---|---|---|
| | 1 | 2 | 3 | |
| **GENERAL SERVICE COST CENTERS** | | | | |
| 1 Capital Related—Bldg & Fixtures | | | | |
| 2 Capital Related—Movable Equip | | | | |
| 3 Plant Operation & Maintenance | | | | |
| 4 Transportation (See Instructions) | | | | |
| 5 Administrative & General | | | | |
| **HHA REIMBURSABLE SERVICES** | | | | |
| 6 Skilled Nursing Care | | | | |
| 7 Physical Therapy | | | | |
| 8 Occupational Therapy | | | | |
| 9 Speech Pathology | | | | |
| 10 Medical Social Services | | | | |
| 11 Home Health Aide | | | | |
| 12 Durable Medical Equipment—Rented | | | | |
| 13 Durable Medical Equipment—Sold | | | | |
| 14 Supplies (See Instructions) | | | | |
| **HHA NONREIMBURSABLE SVCS** | | | | |
| 15 Home Dialysis Aide Services | | | | |
| 16 Respiratory Therapy | | | | |
| 17 Private Duty Nursing | | | | |
| 18 Clinic | | | | |
| 19 Health Promotion Activities | | | | |
| 20 Day Care Program | | | | |
| 21 Home Delivered Meals Program | | | | |
| 22 CORF | | | | |
| **SPECIAL PURPOSE COST CENTER** | | | | |
| 23 Hospice | | | | |
| **OTHER NONREIMBURSABLE COSTS** | | | | |
| 24 Homemaker Service | | | | |
| 25 Other | | | | |
| **OTHER COSTS** | | | | |
| 26 Insurance—Malpractice | | | | |
| 27 Insurance—Other | | | | |
| 28 Interest | | | | |
| 29 TOTAL | | | | |

(1) Transfer the amounts in column 9 to Wkst. A, column 1

FORM HCFA-1728-86 (INSTRUCTIONS FOR THIS WORKSHEET ARE PUBLISHED IN HCFA PUB. 15-11, SEC. 1704) (12-92)

**FIGURE 12.4** Worksheet A-1.

| PROVIDER NO.: | PERIOD: FROM _____ TO _____ | WORKSHEET A–1 | | | |
|---|---|---|---|---|---|
| SUPERVISORS | NURSES | THERAPISTS | AIDES | ALL OTHERS | TOTAL (1) |
| 4 | 5 | 6 | 7 | 8 | 9 |
| | | | | | |
| | | | | | 1 |
| | | | | | 2 |
| | | | | | 3 |
| | | | | | 4 |
| | | | | | 5 |
| | | | | | |
| | | | | | 6 |
| | | | | | 7 |
| | | | | | 8 |
| | | | | | 9 |
| | | | | | 10 |
| | | | | | 11 |
| | | | | | 12 |
| | | | | | 13 |
| | | | | | 14 |
| | | | | | |
| | | | | | 15 |
| | | | | | 16 |
| | | | | | 17 |
| | | | | | 18 |
| | | | | | 19 |
| | | | | | 20 |
| | | | | | 21 |
| | | | | | 22 |
| | | | | | |
| | | | | | 23 |
| | | | | | |
| | | | | | 24 |
| | | | | | 25 |
| | | | | | |
| | | | | | 26 |
| | | | | | 27 |
| | | | | | 28 |
| | | | | | 29 |

## COMPENSATION ANALYSIS
## EMPLOYEE BENEFITS (PAYROLL RELATED)

| | ADMINIS-TRATORS | DIRECTORS | CONSULTANTS | |
|---|---|---|---|---|
| | 1 | 2 | 3 | |
| **GENERAL SERVICE COST CENTERS** | | | | |
| 1 Capital Related—Bldg & Fixtures | | | | |
| 2 Capital Related—Movable Equip | | | | |
| 3 Plant Operation & Maintenance | | | | |
| 4 Transportation (See Instructions) | | | | |
| 5 Administrative & General | | | | |
| **HHA REIMBURSABLE SERVICES** | | | | |
| 6 Skilled Nursing Care | | | | |
| 7 Physical Therapy | | | | |
| 8 Occupational Therapy | | | | |
| 9 Speech Pathology | | | | |
| 10 Medical Social Services | | | | |
| 11 Home Health Aide | | | | |
| 12 Durable Medical Equipment—Rented | | | | |
| 13 Durable Medical Equipment—Sold | | | | |
| 14 Supplies (See Instructions) | | | | |
| **HHA NONREIMBURSABLE SVCS** | | | | |
| 15 Home Dialysis Aide Services | | | | |
| 16 Respiratory Therapy | | | | |
| 17 Private Duty Nursing | | | | |
| 18 Clinic | | | | |
| 19 Health Promotion Activities | | | | |
| 20 Day Care Program | | | | |
| 21 Home Delivered Meals Program | | | | |
| 22 CORF | | | | |
| **SPECIAL PURPOSE COST CENTER** | | | | |
| 23 Hospice | | | | |
| **OTHER NONREIMBURSABLE COSTS** | | | | |
| 24 Homemaker Service | | | | |
| 25 Other | | | | |
| **OTHER COSTS** | | | | |
| 26 Insurance—Malpractice | | | | |
| 27 Insurance—Other | | | | |
| 28 Interest | | | | |
| 29 TOTAL | | | | |

(1) Transfer the amounts in column 9 to Wkst. A, column 2

FORM HCFA-1728-86 (INSTRUCTIONS FOR THIS WORKSHEET ARE PUBLISHED IN HCFA PUB. 15-11, SEC. 1705) (12-92)

**FIGURE 12.5** Worksheet A-2.

| | PROVIDER NO.: | | PERIOD:<br>FROM _____<br>TO _____ | | WORKSHEET A-2 |
|---|---|---|---|---|---|

| SUPERVISORS | NURSES | THERAPISTS | AIDES | ALL OTHERS | TOTAL (1) | |
|---|---|---|---|---|---|---|
| 4 | 5 | 6 | 7 | 8 | 9 | |
| | | | | | | |
| | | | | | | 1 |
| | | | | | | 2 |
| | | | | | | 3 |
| | | | | | | 4 |
| | | | | | | 5 |
| | | | | | | |
| | | | | | | 6 |
| | | | | | | 7 |
| | | | | | | 8 |
| | | | | | | 9 |
| | | | | | | 10 |
| | | | | | | 11 |
| | | | | | | 12 |
| | | | | | | 13 |
| | | | | | | 14 |
| | | | | | | |
| | | | | | | 15 |
| | | | | | | 16 |
| | | | | | | 17 |
| | | | | | | 18 |
| | | | | | | 19 |
| | | | | | | 20 |
| | | | | | | 21 |
| | | | | | | 22 |
| | | | | | | 23 |
| | | | | | | 24 |
| | | | | | | 25 |
| | | | | | | 26 |
| | | | | | | 27 |
| | | | | | | 28 |
| | | | | | | 29 |

COMPENSATION ANALYSIS
CONTRACTED SERVICES/PURCHASED SERVICES

| | | ADMINIS-TRATORS | DIRECTORS | CONSULTANTS | |
|---|---|---|---|---|---|
| | | 1 | 2 | 3 | |
| | **GENERAL SERVICE COST CENTERS** | | | | |
| 1 | Capital Related—Bldg & Fixtures | | | | |
| 2 | Capital Related—Movable Equip | | | | |
| 3 | Plant Operation & Maintenance | | | | |
| 4 | Transportation (See Instructions) | | | | |
| 5 | Administrative & General | | | | |
| | **HHA REIMBURSABLE SERVICES** | | | | |
| 6 | Skilled Nursing Care | | | | |
| 7 | Physical Therapy | | | | |
| 8 | Occupational Therapy | | | | |
| 9 | Speech Pathology | | | | |
| 10 | Medical Social Services | | | | |
| 11 | Home Health Aide | | | | |
| 12 | Durable Medical Equipment—Rented | | | | |
| 13 | Durable Medical Equipment—Sold | | | | |
| 14 | Supplies (See Instructions) | | | | |
| | **HHA NONREIMBURSABLE SVCS** | | | | |
| 15 | Home Dialysis Aide Services | | | | |
| 16 | Respiratory Therapy | | | | |
| 17 | Private Duty Nursing | | | | |
| 18 | Clinic | | | | |
| 19 | Health Promotion Activities | | | | |
| 20 | Day Care Program | | | | |
| 21 | Home Delivered Meals Program | | | | |
| 22 | CORF | | | | |
| | **SPECIAL PURPOSE COST CENTER** | | | | |
| 23 | Hospice | | | | |
| | **OTHER NONREIMBURSABLE COSTS** | | | | |
| 24 | Homemaker Service | | | | |
| 25 | Other | | | | |
| | **OTHER COSTS** | | | | |
| 26 | Insurance—Malpractice | | | | |
| 27 | Insurance—Other | | | | |
| 28 | Interest | | | | |
| 29 | TOTAL | | | | |

(1) Transfer the amounts in column 9 to Wkst. A, column 4

FORM HCFA-1728-86 (INSTRUCTIONS FOR THIS WORKSHEET ARE PUBLISHED IN HCFA PUB. 15-11, SEC. 1706) (12-92)

**FIGURE 12.6** Worksheet A-3.

| | PROVIDER NO.: | | PERIOD:<br>FROM ———————<br>TO ——————— | | WORKSHEET A-3 |
|---|---|---|---|---|---|

| | SUPERVISORS | NURSES | THERAPISTS | AIDES | ALL OTHERS | TOTAL (1) | |
|---|---|---|---|---|---|---|---|
| | 4 | 5 | 6 | 7 | 8 | 9 | |
| | | | | | | | |
| | | | | | | | 1 |
| | | | | | | | 2 |
| | | | | | | | 3 |
| | | | | | | | 4 |
| | | | | | | | 5 |
| | | | | | | | |
| | | | | | | | 6 |
| | | | | | | | 7 |
| | | | | | | | 8 |
| | | | | | | | 9 |
| | | | | | | | 10 |
| | | | | | | | 11 |
| | | | | | | | 12 |
| | | | | | | | 13 |
| | | | | | | | 14 |
| | | | | | | | |
| | | | | | | | 15 |
| | | | | | | | 16 |
| | | | | | | | 17 |
| | | | | | | | 18 |
| | | | | | | | 19 |
| | | | | | | | 20 |
| | | | | | | | 21 |
| | | | | | | | 22 |
| | | | | | | | |
| | | | | | | | 23 |
| | | | | | | | |
| | | | | | | | 24 |
| | | | | | | | 25 |
| | | | | | | | |
| | | | | | | | 26 |
| | | | | | | | 27 |
| | | | | | | | 28 |
| | | | | | | | 29 |

The left margin of each worksheet has a *cost center* designation, or title. A cost center is an agency department or organizational grouping where direct and indirect expenses are accumulated for the services it provides. In the physical therapist salary expense example previously mentioned, the expense would be placed in the *physical therapy* (line 7) cost center of column 5 on Worksheet A-1.

There are twenty-eight cost centers that are classified into six different categories on HCFA-1728. The six categories are

- general service
- home health agency reimbursable services
- home health agency nonreimbursable services
- special purpose cost center
- other nonreimbursable costs
- other costs

General service cost centers are departments or units that render services to parts of, or the entire, agency. These general service cost centers are comprised of the following areas:

- capital-related
- plant operation and maintenance
- transportation
- administration and general (A&G)

Examples of departments that generate general service expense are housekeeping and accounting. The function of these departments is to provide support services to all administrative and clinical departments of the agency. Housekeeping expense would be reported in plant operation and maintenance, and accounting expense would be reported in A&G.

Because general service departments provide services to each other and to clinical disciplines, their costs are reported first. After all other expense is reported in the cost centers, a cost allocation process identifies general service expense that belongs in the proper clinical discipline. This process will be discussed later in the chapter.

The next set of cost centers is the HHA *reimbursable* services. Included in this set are

- skilled nursing care
- physical therapy (PT)
- occupational therapy (OT)
- speech pathology (SP)
- medical social service (MSS)
- home health aide (HHA)
- durable medical equipment (rented and sold) (DME)
- ancillary medical supplies

Within these cost centers are salaries, fringes, contract service, and other expenses applicable to the clinical services reimbursed by M/C. In addition to direct expenses, the appropriate overhead expenses from the general service cost centers are allocated to each reimbursable cost center at this point. Again, the allocation process will be discussed later in the chapter.

The reimbursable cost centers with both direct and overhead expense are the basis for M/C reimbursement. Their expense is transferred to subsequent schedules for final settlement calculations.

In addition to providing M/C reimbursable services, agencies also provide services that are considered nonreimbursable under the home care benefit. The expense for these services is reported in HHA nonreimbursable services, special purpose, and other nonreimbursable cost centers.

The HCFA-1728 has placed the most common nonreimbursable titles in these cost centers. They include

- private duty nursing
- clinic
- home delivered meals program
- Comprehensive Outpatient Rehabilitation Facility (CORF)
- hospice

All of these programs are sponsored by the agency; the programs' direct costs must be reported in a nonreimbursable cost center. The purpose of this reporting requirement is to allocate the appropriate costs from general service cost centers to these programs. This will ensure that general service expense belonging to nonreimbursable cost centers are not improperly allocated to, and included in, reimbursable cost centers.

**Case Study**

An agency sponsoring a hospice will not have a separate finance department for the hospice. The finance department will handle all appropriate functions of the hospice. Therefore, finance department expense reported in A&G must be allocated to all cost centers of the agency, and to the hospice cost center. As explained later in the chapter, the reporting of direct expense in the hospice cost center will ensure the hospice receives its fair percentage of finance department expense.

## Medicare Reimbursed Noncertified Programs

The direct and allocated general service costs of the CORF and hospice cost centers are the starting point for M/C reimbursement under separate, respective cost reporting mechanisms. These costs are transferred to another cost report in accordance with prescribed M/C regulations, and will not be further considered in the determination of the certified agency's reimbursable costs.

## Grant and Special Fund Expense

The reporting of grant or special funds expense is always a concern in the cost reporting process.

**Case Study**

An agency may receive a $10,000 grant to provide for nonreimbursable or uncovered items such as dentures or eyeglasses.

The agency will incur $10,000 in expense for providing the items. The grant is used solely for care, equipment, or service to the patient; none of the funds are spent on administration of the grant. One may reasonably assume that the revenue and expense is offset and has no effect on M/C reimbursement. The FI takes a different approach to the reporting of the expense. They reason that the grant expense should be reported in a nonreimbursable cost center for purposes of receiving allocated general service expense.

Since the grant requires accounting, purchasing, and other services, these expenses should be allocated to the $10,000 in direct grant expense. This has the negative effect of reducing general service cost center expense, therefore reducing M/C reimbursable costs.

### Other Costs

Other costs make up the final set of cost centers, including *insurance—malpractice, insurance—other,* and *interest.* These cost centers were established for the purpose of separately identifying reimbursable insurance and interest costs. They are then reclassified to general service cost centers for proper allocation to all cost centers.

## Reclassification and Adjustment of Expenses

Expenses classified in cost centers of all worksheets are reported from the general ledger, or *expense accounts* of the *trial balance of expenses.* Certain expense may be erroneously posted to an expense account, or expense may be posted in the correct account for accounting purposes but may be inappropriate for M/C cost reporting purposes.

These problems can be corrected on *Worksheet A-4, Reclassifications.* This reporting form allows for the identification of cost that is not properly reported in its correct cost center, and for the reclassification of that expense.

As mentioned previously, both insurance and interest expense are reclassified from individual cost centers to general service cost centers. This reclassification is reported on Worksheet A-4 as well.

Figure 12.7 is a reproduction detailing Worksheet A-4.

The last component of reporting expense is to make any necessary adjustments in accordance with M/C regulations. This is accomplished on *Worksheet A-5, Adjustments to Expenses* and is represented in Figure 12.8.

As detailed in Chapter 11, certain income or rebates must be applied to reduce the associated expense. This reduction is reported on Worksheet A-5.

A freestanding agency may have a parent or other similar oversight organization. The related organization may have incurred expense in providing services to the freestanding agency. Proper and reasonable expense for such services may be included on the agency's cost report. The addition of expense is reported on Worksheet A-5.

If the FI audit finds expense that is not proper and reasonable, a disallowance of expense will be reported on Worksheet A-5. Thus Worksheet A-5 is used by both the agency and the FI to adjust expense.

## Cost Allocation

Upon completion of Worksheets A-1 through A-5, the classifications, reclassifications, and adjustments of expense are transferred to Worksheet A (Figure 12.3). The final column on Worksheet A is the net expense for cost allocation.

### Worksheet B

Costs from the general service cost centers, such as A&G, are now ready to be allocated to all other cost centers. *Worksheet B, Cost Allocation—General Service Cost* is the schedule where the actual allocation takes place. An example of Worksheet B is found in Figure 12.9.

The allocation process is termed the *step-down method*. Step-down first allocates, or passes down, the expense of the general service cost center that services the greatest number of other cost centers. The next cost center to be *stepped-down* is the one that is second in servicing all other cost centers. This process continues until the last cost center, which services the least number of other cost centers, is allocated.

Worksheet B is designed so the general service cost centers are the titles of its columns. The rows are the same as in previous worksheets. The hierarchy of general service cost centers to be allocated after net expense, and the order of column titles is

- capital related cost—building and fixtures
- capital related cost—moveable equipment
- plant operation and maintenance
- transportation
- A&G

General service expense from one cost center may be allocated to another general service cost center. This expense will be reallocated as the step-down process continues.

### Worksheet B-1

The step-down method utilizes statistics for the allocation process. Used in this context, statistics means values applied in the mathematical allocation of general service expense. The statistics are reported on *Worksheet B-1, Cost Allocation—Statistical Basis*.

Figure 12.10 is a reproduction of Worksheet B-1.

Statistics required for general service cost center allocations by the FI are *square feet* for capital and maintenance, *mileage* for transportation, and *net (accumulated) cost* for A&G.

Square feet is the actual square footage of the facility where the agency operates. Square footage includes all rental and depreciation expense for space. The expense is identified with useable and common space (such as corridors, building mechanical rooms, etc.). The cost of common space is factored into useable space. Mileage is the distance driven by agency personnel while conducting agency business. Accumulated cost is the total direct expense, per cost center, reported in Worksheet A after reclassifications and adjustments.

The mathematics of step-down apportion each general service's cost to all other cost centers.

## RECLASSIFICATIONS

| EXPLANATION OF RECLASSIFICATION ENTRY | CODE (1) | COST CENTER | |
|---|---|---|---|
| | 1 | 2 | |
| 1 | | | |
| 2 | | | |
| 3 | | | |
| 4 | | | |
| 5 | | | |
| 6 | | | |
| 7 | | | |
| 8 | | | |
| 9 | | | |
| 10 | | | |
| 11 | | | |
| 12 | | | |
| 13 | | | |
| 14 | | | |
| 15 | | | |
| 16 | | | |
| 17 | | | |
| 18 | | | |
| 19 | | | |
| 20 | | | |
| 21 | | | |
| 22 | | | |
| 23 | | | |
| 24 | | | |
| 25 | | | |
| 26 | | | |
| 27 | | | |
| 28 | | | |
| 29 | | | |
| 30 | | | |
| 31 | | | |
| 32 | | | |
| 33 | | | |
| 34 | | | |
| 35 | | | |
| 36 | TOTAL RECLASSIFICATIONS (Sum of col. 4 must equal sum of col. 7) | | |

(1)  A letter (A, B, etc) must be entered on each line to identify each reclassification entry.

(2)  Transfer to Worksheet A, column 7, line as appropriate.

FORM HCFA-1728-86 (INSTRUCTIONS FOR THIS WORKSHEET ARE PUBLISHED IN HCFA PUB. 15-11, SEC. 1707) (12-92)

**FIGURE 12.7** Worksheet A-4.

| | PROVIDER NO.: | PERIOD:<br>FROM ———————————<br>TO ——————————— | | | WORKSHEET A–4 |
|---|---|---|---|---|---|

| INCREASE | | DECREASE | | | |
|---|---|---|---|---|---|
| LINE NO. | AMOUNT (2) | COST CENTER | LINE NO. | AMOUNT (2) | |
| 3 | 4 | 5 | 6 | 7 | |
| | | | | | |
| | | | | | |
| | | | | | |
| | | | | | |
| | | | | | |
| | | | | | |
| | | | | | |
| | | | | | |
| | | | | | |
| | | | | | |
| | | | | | |
| | | | | | |
| | | | | | |
| | | | | | |
| | | | | | |
| | | | | | |
| | | | | | |
| | | | | | |
| | | | | | |
| | | | | | |
| | | | | | |
| | | | | | |
| | | | | | |
| | | | | | |
| | | | | | |
| | | | | | |
| | | | | | |
| | | | | | |
| | | | | | |
| | | | | | |
| | | | | | |
| | | | | | |
| | | | | | |
| | | | | | |
| | | | | | |

**ADJUSTMENTS TO EXPENSES**

PROVIDER NO.:

PERIOD:
FROM _____
TO _____

WORKSHEET A-5

| | Description (1) | Basis for Adjustment(s) 1 | Amount 2 | Expense Classification on Worksheet A | |
|---|---|---|---|---|---|
| | | | | Cost Center 3 | Line No. 4 |
| 1 | Excess Funds Generated From Operations, Other Than Net Income | B | | | |
| 2 | Trade, Quantity, Time and Other Discounts on Purchases (Chap. 8) | B | | | |
| 3 | Rebates and Refunds of Expenses (Chap. 8) | B | | | |
| 4 | Home Office Costs (Chap. 21) | A | | | |
| 5 | Adjustments resulting from transaction with related organization (Chap. 10) | Fr Wks A-6 | | | |
| 6 | Sale of Medical Records and Abstracts | B | | | |
| 7 | Income from Imposition of interest, finance or penalty charges (Chap. 21) | B | | | |
| 8 | Sale of medical and surgical supplies to other than patients | A | | | |
| 9 | Sale of Drugs to other than patients | A | | | |

| | Description | Fr Supp Wks A–8–3 | | | | | | | | |
|---|---|---|---|---|---|---|---|---|---|---|
| 10 | Physical therapy adjustment (Chap. 14) | | | | | | | | | |
| 11 | Interest expense on Medicare overpayments and borrowings to repay Medicare overpayments | A | | | | | | | | |
| 12 | | | | | | | | | | |
| 13 | | | | | | | | | | |
| 14 | | | | | | | | | | |
| 15 | | | | | | | | | | |
| 16 | | | | | | | | | | |
| 17 | | | | | | | | | | |
| 18 | | | | | | | | | | |
| 19 | | | | | | | | | | |
| 20 | | | | | | | | | | |
| 21 | TOTAL (Sum of lines 1–20) | | | | | | | | | |

(1) Description—All line references in this column pertain to the Provider Reimbursement Manual, Part I.

(2) Basis for adjustment (SEE INSTRUCTIONS)
  A. Costs—If cost, including applicable overhead, can be determined
  B. Amount Received—If cost cannot be determined

FORM HCFA-172886 (INSTRUCTIONS FOR THIS WORKSHEET ARE PUBLISHED IN HCFA PUB. 15-11, SEC. 1708) (12–92)

**FIGURE 12.8** Worksheet A-5.

## COST ALLOCATION—GENERAL SERVICE COST

| | COST CENTER | NET EXPENSE FOR COST ALLOCATION (FR WKST A) | CAP REL COST BUILDING & FIXTURES | |
|---|---|---|---|---|
| | | 0 | 1 | |
| | **GENERAL SERVICE COST CENTERS** | | | |
| 1 | Capital Related—Bldg & Fixtures | | | |
| 2 | Capital Related—Movable Equipment | | | |
| 3 | Plant Operation and Maintenance | | | |
| 4 | Transportation (See Instructions) | | | |
| 5 | Administrative and General | | | |
| | **HHA REIMBURSABLE SERVICES** | | | |
| 6 | Skilled Nursing Care | | | |
| 7 | Physical Therapy | | | |
| 8 | Occupational Therapy | | | |
| 9 | Speech Pathology | | | |
| 10 | Medical Social Services | | | |
| 11 | Home Health Aide | | | |
| 12 | Durable Medical Equipment—Rented | | | |
| 13 | Durable Medical Equipment—Sold | | | |
| 14 | Supplies (See Instructions) | | | |
| | **HHA NONREIMBURSABLE SERVICES** | | | |
| 15 | Home Dialysis Aide Services | | | |
| 16 | Respiratory Therapy | | | |
| 17 | Private Duty Nursing | | | |
| 18 | Clinic | | | |
| 19 | Health Promotion Activities | | | |
| 20 | Day Care Program | | | |
| 21 | Home Delivered Meals Program | | | |
| 22 | CORF | | | |
| | **SPECIAL PURPOSE COST CENTER** | | | |
| 23 | Hospice | | | |
| | **OTHER NONREIMBURSABLE COSTS** | | | |
| 24 | Homemaker Service | | | |
| 25 | Other | | | |
| 26 | | | | |
| 27 | | | | |
| 28 | | | | |
| 29 | TOTAL | | | |

FORM HCFA-1728-86 (INSTRUCTIONS FOR THIS WORKSHEET ARE PUBLISHED IN HCFA PUB. 15-11, SEC. 1709) (12-92)

**FIGURE 12.9** Worksheet B.

| PROVIDER NO.: | PERIOD:<br>FROM ————————————<br>TO ———————————— | | | WORKSHEET B |
|---|---|---|---|---|
| **CAP REL<br>COST<br>MOVABLE<br>EQUIPMENT** | **PLANT<br>OPERATION<br>MAINTENANCE** | **TRANS-<br>PORTATION** | **ADMINISTRA-<br>TIVE AND<br>GENERAL** | **TOTAL** |
| **2** | **3** | **4** | **5** | **6** |
| | | | | | 1 |
| | | | | | 2 |
| | | | | | 3 |
| | | | | | 4 |
| | | | | | 5 |
| | | | | | 6 |
| | | | | | 7 |
| | | | | | 8 |
| | | | | | 9 |
| | | | | | 10 |
| | | | | | 11 |
| | | | | | 12 |
| | | | | | 13 |
| | | | | | 14 |
| | | | | | 15 |
| | | | | | 16 |
| | | | | | 17 |
| | | | | | 18 |
| | | | | | 19 |
| | | | | | 20 |
| | | | | | 21 |
| | | | | | 22 |
| | | | | | 23 |
| | | | | | 24 |
| | | | | | 25 |
| | | | | | 26 |
| | | | | | 27 |
| | | | | | 28 |
| | | | | | 29 |

## COST ALLOCATION—STATISTICAL BASIS

| COST CENTER | | CAP REL COST BUILDING & FIXTURES (Square Feet) | |
|---|---|---|---|
| | 0 | 1 | |
| **GENERAL SERVICE COST CENTERS** | | | |
| 1 Capital Related—Bldg & Fixtures | | | |
| 2 Capital Related—Movable Equipment | | | |
| 3 Plant Operation and Maintenance | | | |
| 4 Transportation (See Instructions) | | | |
| 5 Administrative and General | | | |
| **HHA REIMBURSABLE SERVICES** | | | |
| 6 Skilled Nursing Care | | | |
| 7 Physical Therapy | | | |
| 8 Occupational Therapy | | | |
| 9 Speech Pathology | | | |
| 10 Medical Social Services | | | |
| 11 Home Health Aide | | | |
| 12 Durable Medical Equipment—Rented | | | |
| 13 Durable Medical Equipment—Sold | | | |
| 14 Supplies (See Instructions) | | | |
| **HHA NONREIMBURSABLE SERVICES** | | | |
| 15 Home Dialysis Aide Services | | | |
| 16 Respiratory Therapy | | | |
| 17 Private Duty Nursing | | | |
| 18 Clinic | | | |
| 19 Health Promotion Activities | | | |
| 20 Day Care Program | | | |
| 21 Home Delivered Meals Program | | | |
| 22 CORF | | | |
| **SPECIAL PURPOSE COST CENTER** | | | |
| 23 Hospice | | | |
| **OTHER NONREIMBURSABLE COSTS** | | | |
| 24 Homemaker Service | | | |
| 25 Other | | | |
| 26 | | | |
| 27 | | | |
| 28 | | | |
| 29 Cost to be Allocated (Per Wkst B) | | | |
| 30 Unit Cost Multiplier | | | |

FORM HCFA-1728-86 (INSTRUCTIONS FOR THIS WORKSHEET ARE PUBLISHED IN HCFA PUB. 15-11, SEC. 1709) (12-92)

**FIGURE 12.10** Worksheet B-1.

| PROVIDER NO.: | | PERIOD: FROM ——————— TO ——————— | | WORKSHEET B-1 |
|---|---|---|---|---|
| **CAP REL COST MOVABLE EQUIPMENT (Square Ft or $ Value)** | **PLANT OPERATION MAINTENANCE (Square Feet)** | **TRANS-PORTATION (Mileage)** | **ADMINISTRA-TIVE AND GENERAL (Net Cost Col 0, Wkst B)** | |
| 2 | 3 | 4 | 5 | 6 |
| | | | | |
| | | | | 1 |
| | | | | 2 |
| | | | | 3 |
| | | | | 4 |
| | | | | 5 |
| | | | | |
| | | | | 6 |
| | | | | 7 |
| | | | | 8 |
| | | | | 9 |
| | | | | 10 |
| | | | | 11 |
| | | | | 12 |
| | | | | 13 |
| | | | | 14 |
| | | | | |
| | | | | 15 |
| | | | | 16 |
| | | | | 17 |
| | | | | 18 |
| | | | | 19 |
| | | | | 20 |
| | | | | 21 |
| | | | | 22 |
| | | | | |
| | | | | 23 |
| | | | | |
| | | | | 24 |
| | | | | 25 |
| | | | | 26 |
| | | | | 27 |
| | | | | 28 |
| | | | | 29 |
| | | | | 30 |

For example, an agency may have 20,000 square feet in its facility. Approximately 4,000 square feet is devoted to direct care nursing. In this example 20 percent (4,000 divided by 20,000) of capital expense would be allocated to the skilled nursing care cost center.

Accurately compiling and maintaining Worksheet B-1 statistics is critical. Since general service cost is a sizable portion of total expense, it is important that the statistics properly step-down the cost to reimbursable and nonreimbursable cost centers. Also, the statistics are examined by the FI on audit of the cost report.

## Apportionment of Patient Service Costs

The next step in the cost report is to transfer HHA reimbursable services cost centers from Worksheet B to *Worksheet C, Apportionment of Patient Service Costs*. At this point all other expense applicable to nonreimbursable cost centers are eliminated in the calculation of M/C reimbursement. Figure 12.11 is a reproduction of Worksheet C.

Worksheet C is divided into two categories—visit services and other services. Visit services include nursing, therapy, medical social service, and home health aide cost centers. Other services include home medical equipment (HME) and ancillary medical supply cost centers.

Visit service expense for each discipline is first divided by total visits of the discipline to determine a cost per visit. The cost per visit is then multiplied by actual M/C visits made by the discipline to calculate M/C cost. This process is known as apportioning out M/C expense from total expense. The M/C cost for each discipline is then totaled to determine aggregate M/C cost for visit services.

### Case Study
A skilled nursing cost center is as follows.
1. there are total direct and allocated expenses of $900,000 (recorded on Worksheet C, column 2, line 1)
2. total visits are 10,000 (column 3)
3. M/C visits are 6,000 (column 5)
4. the total expense of $900,000 is then divided by total visits of 10,000 to report a cost per visit of $90 in column 4
5. the cost per visit of $90 is then multiplied by M/C visits of 6,000 to calculate M/C reimbursement of $540,000 in column 8

The M/C cost from visit services are then subjected to *routine cost limits* for each service. The limits, commonly known as caps, are promulgated annually by the Health Care Financing Administration (HCFA) through analysis of national labor and nonlabor components of visit services. The labor portion is then adjusted by the FIs to account for regional differences in wages.

Caps are promulgated for cost reporting periods beginning July 1 of every year and are adjusted for reporting periods beginning August 1 through June 1 of the subsequent year. Therefore an agency with a cost reporting period beginning January 1 will receive caps adjusted for inflation occurring between July 1 and December 31.

Individual discipline caps are multiplied by M/C visits to determine the maximum amount allowed for M/C reimbursement. The individual caps are then totaled to determine the aggregate cap of M/C reimbursement. The M/C calculation of reimbursement for visit services then requires a comparison of aggregate M/C cost to aggregate caps. The lower of cost or caps is then carried forward in the reimbursement calculation.

**Case Study**
Referring to the previous skilled nursing example, the $540,000 will be compared to a cap. If the cap for the agency is equal to or greater than $90 per visit, then the agency will receive the full $540,000 in M/C reimbursement. If the cost per visit is greater than the cap, then the agency may have a reduction of M/C reimbursable skilled nursing expense. An $80 cap, for instance, would result in a reduction of $10 per visit from the calculated cost per visit of $90. The $10 multiplied by 6,000 M/C visits would result in a total amount subject to reduction of $60,000.

To avoid the $60,000 reduction the agency would need to have one of the other five disciplines *under* its respective cap by $60,000 or more. Comparing disciplines in the aggregate affords an agency to offset reimbursement reductions in higher cost disciplines by providing other services that are under caps.

The second component of Worksheet C is to apportion the M/C cost of HME and supplies. Similar to the visit disciplines, the expense in these cost centers is apportioned by dividing total charges for each cost center to determine a cost per charge. The cost per charge is then multiplied by M/C charges to determine M/C cost. Unlike visit services, HME and supplies are not subject to caps.

## Calculation of Reimbursement Settlement

After the apportionment of expense, M/C visit and other services reimbursement is carried forward to *Worksheet D, Calculation of Reimbursement Settlement*. Please refer to Figure 12.12 for the detail of Worksheet D.

This HCFA form compares M/C reimbursable cost to M/C charges for services rendered under the lower of cost or charge (LCC) provision described in Chapter 11.

After the LCC comparison is made, the lower of M/C cost or charges may be subject to other computations. These computations result from unusual reimbursement situations such as the disposition of major assets. Because they occur infrequently, they will not be discussed in this text. The reader is directed to the *Medicare Reimbursement Manual HCFA-Pub. 15–1*.

The final M/C reimbursement is then compared to what was paid by the FI during the agency's billing time period. If M/C reimbursable cost is higher than FI interim payments, a receivable occurs and the FI issues a final payment. The opposite situation results in a payable and the agency is required to issue a payment to the FI.

APPORTIONMENT OF PATIENT SERVICE COSTS
(For Cost Reporting Periods
Beginning on or After July 1, 1986)

COMPUTATION OF THE LESSER OF AGGREGATE MEDICARE COST OR THE AGGREGATE OF THE MEDICARE LIMITATION

| Cost Per Visit Computation | From Wkst B, Col. 6, Line: | Total | | Average Cost Per Visit (Cols 2 ÷ 3) |
|---|---|---|---|---|
| Patient Services | | Cost | Visits | |
| | 1 | 2 | 3 | 4 |
| 1 Skilled Nursing | 6 | | | |
| 2 Physical Therapy | 7 | | | |
| 3 Occupational Therapy | 8 | | | |
| 4 Speech Pathology | 9 | | | |
| 5 Medical Social Services | 10 | | | |
| 6 Home Health Aide Services | 11 | | | |
| 7 Total (Sum of lines 1-6) | | | | |

| Cost Limitation Computation | | | | Program Cost Limits |
|---|---|---|---|---|
| Patient Services | | | | |
| | 1 | 2 | 3 | 4 |
| 8 Skilled Nursing | | | | |
| 9 Physical Therapy | | | | |
| 10 Occupational Therapy | | | | |
| 11 Speech Pathology | | | | |
| 12 Medical Social Services | | | | |
| 13 Home Health Aide Services | | | | |
| 14 Total (Sum of lines 8-13) | | | | |

| Supplies and Equipment Cost Computations | From Wkst B, Col. 6, Line: | Total Cost | Total Charges from HHA Record | Ratio (Col 2 ÷ 3) |
|---|---|---|---|---|
| Other Patient Services | | | | |
| | 1 | 2 | 3 | 4 |
| 15 Cost of DME Rented (See Instructions) | 12 | | | |
| 16 Cost of DME Sold (See Instructions) | 13 | | | |
| 17 Cost of Medical Supplies | 14 | | | |

FORM HCFA-1728-91 (12-92) (INSTRUCTIONS FOR THIS WORKSHEET ARE PUBLISHED IN HCFA PUB. 15-11, SEC. 1711–1711.2)

**FIGURE 12.11** Worksheet C.

| PROVIDER NO.: | PERIOD: FROM _____ TO _____ | WORKSHEET C |
| --- | --- | --- |

| | Medicare Program Visits | | | Cost of Medicare Services | | | Total | |
| --- | --- | --- | --- | --- | --- | --- | --- | --- |
| | Part A | Part B | Other Part B | Part A (Col. 4 x 5) | Part B (Col. 4 x 6) | Other pt. B (Col. 4 x 7) | (Sum of Cols 8, 9 & 10) | |
| | 5 | 6 | 7 | 8 | 9 | 10 | 11 | |
| | | | | | | | | 1 |
| | | | | | | | | 2 |
| | | | | | | | | 3 |
| | | | | | | | | 4 |
| | | | | | | | | 5 |
| | | | | | | | | 6 |
| | | | | | | | | 7 |

| | Medicare Program Visits | | | Cost of Medicare Services | | | Total | |
| --- | --- | --- | --- | --- | --- | --- | --- | --- |
| | Part A | Part B | Other Part B | Part A (Col. 4 x 5) | Part B (Col. 4 x 6) | Other pt. B (Col. 4 x 7) | (Sum of Cols 8, 9 & 10) | |
| | 5 | 6 | 7 | 8 | 9 | 10 | 11 | |
| | | | | | | | | 8 |
| | | | | | | | | 9 |
| | | | | | | | | 10 |
| | | | | | | | | 11 |
| | | | | | | | | 12 |
| | | | | | | | | 13 |
| | | | | | | | | 14 |

| | Medicare Covered Charges | | | Cost of Services | | | | |
| --- | --- | --- | --- | --- | --- | --- | --- | --- |
| | Part A | Part B | Other Part B | Part A (Col. 4 x 5) | Part B (Col. 4 x 6) | Other pt. B (Col. 4 x 7) | | |
| | 5 | 6 | 7 | 8 | 9 | 10 | | |
| | | | | | | | | 15 |
| | | | | | | | | 16 |
| | | | | | | | | 17 |

# CALCULATION OF REIMBURSEMENT SETTLEMENT PART A AND PART B SERVICES

PROVIDER NO.: _____

PERIOD: FROM _____ TO _____

WORKSHEET D
PART I & II

## PART I—COMPUTATION OF THE LESSER OF REASONABLE COST OR CUSTOMARY CHARGES

| | Description | PART A | | PART B | | |
|---|---|---|---|---|---|---|
| | | Other Than DME | DME | Other Than DME | DME | Other Services |
| | | 1 | 2 | 3 | 4 | 5 |
| 1 | Reasonable Cost of Title XVIII Part A & Part B Services | | | | | |
| 2 | Reasonable Cost of Services (See Instructions) | | | | | |
| 3 | Primary payor amounts | | | | | |
| 4 | Net cost (Line 1 minus line 2) | | | | | |
| 5 | Allowable return on equity capital (From Supp. Wkst. F–3, Part III, col. 2, lines 1–4) | | | | | |
| 6 | Total reasonable cost (Line 1 plus line 4) | | | | | |
| | Total charges for title XVIII – Part A & Part B Services | | | | | |
| | Customary Charges | | | | | |
| 7 | Amount actually collected from patients liable for payment for services on a charge basis (From your records) | | | | | |
| 8 | Amount that would have been realized from patients liable for payment for services on a charge basis had such payment been made in accordance with 42 CFR 413.13(b) | | | | | |
| 9 | Ratio of line 7 to 8 (Not to exceed 1.0000) | | | | | |
| 10 | Total customary charges—title XVIII (Multiply line 9 x line 6 each column) | | | | | |
| 11 | Excess of total customary charges over total reasonable cost (Complete only if line 10 exceeds line 5) | | | | | |
| 12 | Excess of reasonable cost over customary Charges (Complete if line 5 exceeds line 10) | | | | | |

170

PART II—COMPUTATION OF REIMBURSEMENT SETTLEMENT

| | Description | Part A Services 1 | Part B Services 2 | Other Services 3 |
|---|---|---|---|---|
| 13 | Total reasonable cost (See Instructions) | | | |
| 14 | Part B deductibles billed to Medicare patients (exclude coinsurance) | | | |
| 15 | Subtotal (Line 13 minus lines 14) | | | |
| 16 | Excess reasonable cost (from line 12) | | | |
| 17 | Subtotal (Line 15 minus line 16) | | | |
| 18 | Coinsurance billed to Medicare patients (From your records) | | | |
| 19 | Net cost (Line 17 minus line 18) | | | |
| 20 | Reimbursable bad debts (From your records) | | | |
| 21 | Total Costs—Current cost reporting period (See Instructions) | | | |
| 22 | Recovery of unreimbursed cost under lesser of reasonable cost or customary charges (From Supp Wkst D–2, Part II, line 9, columns 1 and 2) | | | |
| 23 | Amounts applicable to prior cost reporting periods resulting from disposition of depreciable assets | | | |
| 24 | Recovery of excess depreciation resulting from agencies' termination or decrease in Medicare utilization | | | |
| 25 | Unrefunded charges to beneficiaries for excess costs erroneously collected based on correction of cost limit | | | |
| 26A | Total cost before sequestration—(Sum of lines 21 and 22 plus/minus line 23 minus sum of lines 24 and 25) | | | |
| 26B | Sequestration Adjustment (See Instructions) | | | |
| 26C | Amount reimbursable after sequestration adjustment (Line 26A minus line 26B) | | | |
| 27 | Total interim payments (From Worksheet D–1, line 4) | | | |
| 28 | Balance due HHA/Medicare program (Line 26C minus line 27) (Indicate overpayments in brackets) | | | |
| 29 | Protested amounts (nonallowable cost report items) in accordance with HCFA Pub. 15–11, section 115.2(B) | | | |
| 30 | Balance due HHA/Medicare program (Line 28 plus or minus line 29) (Indicate overpayments in brackets) | | | |

FORM HCFA-1728-91 (12-92)  (INSTRUCTIONS FOR THIS WORKSHEET ARE PUBLISHED IN HCFA  PUB. 15-11, SEC. 1712–1712.2)

**FIGURE 12.12** Worksheet D.

171

## Other Worksheets

There are other worksheets required by the FI that pertain to the agency's balance sheet and income statement. These worksheets do not have a direct effect on the calculation of M/C reimbursable cost.

Additionally, FIs may require questionnaires to be completed and submitted with the cost report. These questionnaires request information on agency financial policies and procedures. The FI may also request salary and compensation package information on senior-level management positions.

# HOSPITAL-BASED MEDICARE COST REPORTS

A hospital-based agency is considered a department of the hospital for hospital M/C cost report purposes. Therefore the agency cost centers that are on the freestanding cost report are also reported on the hospital cost report along with the hospital's other cost centers.

As with a freestanding agency cost report, the hospital cost report has classification, reclassification, and adjustment of expense for all its departments, including the agency. This leads to the expense of hospital general service cost centers being allocated to agency general service and reimbursable cost centers. The overall hospital allocation process is identical to the freestanding agency cost report with the exception that more cost centers are involved.

To properly identify the hospital-based agency cost data, the hospital cost report has a separate set of schedules, *Supplemental Worksheet H.* These schedules pertain solely to the agency as a department of the hospital.

The format of these schedules is similar to the HCFA-1728 with one exception. The general service section is limited to one cost center, *Administrative and General—HHA.* All hospital capital, interest, and other administrative and general items are allocated to this cost center.

*Supplemental Worksheet H-4* then takes the A&G cost center and reallocates all expense to the cost centers within the agency. These cost centers with direct and overhead costs go through the apportionment and final settlement processes similar to the HCFA-1728.

# FILING DEADLINES

Medicare cost reports for freestanding agencies and hospitals are required to be filed ninety calendar days after the close of a fiscal year (FY). Therefore, an agency or hospital with a FY ending December 31 has a filing deadline of April 1 of the next year.

Agencies may request in writing a deadline extension for valid circumstances. An example of a valid circumstance might be that the agency had difficulty finalizing its certified financial statements and reporting expense. In this instance the FI may grant the extension, usually for thirty days. The FI may extend the filing deadline in instances where the FI is aware of circumstances that will affect many providers in obtaining final cost report data.

## CONCLUSION

The completion of the annual cost report is a mandatory requirement for agencies to participate in the M/C program. The report summarizes expense and statistics to determine the cost per visit for six disciplines. Expense is then compared to both caps and charges, and the lower of the three is final reimbursable cost.

Completion of an interim cost report on a monthly or quarterly basis provides an agency with a current estimate of the M/C payment rate and reimbursable expense. It also serves as a useful management tool, providing individual cost per visit information for each discipline. These results will give agency management an indicator of financial status and allow for any immediate action to avoid a year-end negative financial impact.

### *Suggested Reading*

U.S. Department of Health and Human Services Health Care Financing Administration. (1994). *Medicare Provider Reimbursement Manual HCFA-Pub. 15–1.* Chapters 23 and 24.

U.S. Department of Health and Human Services Health Care Financing Administration. (1994). *Medicare Provider Reimbursement Manual HCFA-Pub. 15–II.* Sections 1701 through 1713.

# CHAPTER

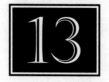

# 13

# Medicare Payment for Provider Services

**Timothy Riordan**

Chapter 11 provided a general overview of how Medicare (M/C) reimbursement is determined for agency services. At this point, a description of how actual monetary payment for services is made is appropriate. Without an adequate and timely revenue stream, an agency will find itself hard-pressed to meet monetary liabilities such as salaries and operating expenses.

Rate calculations, payment systems, and billing process are the mechanisms by which the fiscal intermediary (FI) provides the revenue stream to the agency. In this chapter the acronym FI is the generic descriptor for the regional home health intermediary (RHHI). The fundamentals of rate calculations, payment systems, and the billing process will be discussed in this chapter.

# DETERMINATION OF THE PAYMENT RATE

The FI must calculate a payment rate for agency services rendered to M/C beneficiaries. The M/C cost report is the best source of information for rate calculation.

The annual reimbursement is found in detail on the final settlement pages of the M/C cost report *HCFA-1728, Worksheets C* and *D* (see Figures 12.11 and 12.12, respectively). Final settlement is the determination and reconciliation of M/C reimbursable cost and total payments for an annual time period. The difference between cost and payments is remitted to either the provider or FI in the final settlement. These schedules provide M/C cost, routine cost limits or caps, charges, and visits necessary for the calculation.

The FI reviews M/C cost, caps, and charges, and similar to the final settlement, takes the lower of the three as reimbursement for services. This number is then divided by M/C visits reported on Worksheet C to determine the cost or payment per visit for M/C services.

An example will be helpful. The annual M/C reimbursable cost for a particular agency is $1 million for 10,000 M/C visits provided. In this example both charges and caps are in excess of reimbursable cost. The payment rate is then determined by calculating $1 million divided by 10,000 M/C visits for a $100 per visit cost.

## Average Cost per Visit

It should be noted that this methodology results in one *average cost per visit* rate for all services. Therefore each visit billed to the FI, whether skilled nursing, physical therapy, or home health aide, will be paid at the same rate.

This calculated average payment rate does not allow for a separate payment for ancillary medical supplies or home medical equipment (HME) provided to patients. Ancillary medical supplies are nonroutine items, as defined by Medicare regulations, used in the provision of patient care. Examples include bedpans, catheters, and cotton dressings. In determining the total payment rate for all services, an additional payment amount per visit is calculated to account for ancillary medical supplies. Home medical equipment reimbursement is provided for under a separate M/C fee schedule.

## Trending

Cost report information utilized by the FI may not be current for the rate year under review. The FI relies on the latest cost report filed and, if necessary, will utilize trend factors to update the rate from the cost report year to the current year.

The FI may employ its own self-defined *safety factor* on the calculated payment rate. The FI will reduce the payment rate by a small percentage to avoid overpayment in case the final reimbursable cost per visit decreases. A decrease in cost per visit may result from expense disallowances during an FI audit or from an increase in agency visit volume.

Conversely, an agency that is over the caps or has a lower of cost or charge problem (LCC) should not have a safety factor imposed. Expense disallowances or increases in agency visit volume will not affect the rate being held to caps or charges.

During the course of its fiscal year (FY), the agency should periodically perform calculations of the M/C payment rate. If the calculations vary materially from the promulgated rate, the FI should be requested to revise the rate. This should avoid large overpayments or underpayments that may have a negative impact on cash flow.

# PAYMENT METHODOLOGIES

After a M/C payment rate is set, there are two methodologies by which an agency will receive cash—*interim payments* and *settlements*.

## Interim Payments

Interim payments are made to the agency during the course of the billing year for M/C services provided. The FI offers two forms of payments—*nonperiodic interim payment* (Non-PIP) and *periodic interim payment* (PIP).

### Nonperiodic Interim Payment

Non-PIP is payment for approved visits. If an agency bills 100 visits, the FI will issue a payment for 100 visits multiplied by the single visit payment rate.

This type of payment system is very simple, but may cause erratic cash flow. Agencies experiencing difficulties in submitting bills to the FI will lose the opportunity to gain money or interest savings. Agencies under non-PIP that experience a period of growth will not receive adequate cash to sustain such growth and meet incurred financial obligations associated with growth.

### Periodic Interim Payment

To alleviate such problems, M/C instituted the PIP system. Under PIP, an agency receives a biweekly check for the reimbursement of anticipated services rendered. It does not matter how many visits are billed during the time period; the agency will receive a check for a predetermined amount every two weeks.

To calculate PIP reimbursement, the FI must determine an agency's expected annual reimbursement by first promulgating a payment rate. Then the FI forecasts an annual M/C visit volume. The volume number is determined by utilizing agency historical data and perhaps the agency's current forecast figures.

Next, the FI multiplies the payment rate by the volume number to calculate annual reimbursement. Last, the annual reimbursement is divided by twenty-six annual biweekly time periods to determine the PIP amount.

To illustrate PIP calculation, the following example is offered. An agency with a M/C payment rate of $100 per visit has a forecasted annual volume of 52,000 M/C visits. Multiply $100 per visit by 52,000 visits and divide by 26 for a biweekly PIP check of $200,000.

The PIP methodology requires an agency to constantly monitor its M/C visit volume. Any increase or decrease in volume could result in a significant M/C receivable or payable. Certain intermediaries require agencies to report visit volume monthly or quarterly to ensure the annual reimbursement is accurate.

Usually there are more overpayments than underpayments when the PIP methodology is utilized. Therefore the FI establishes criteria for an agency to maintain its PIP status.

First, the agency must have an appreciable number of M/C reimbursement payments during the FY. Most FIs consider an annual M/C reimbursement of $100,000 as appreciable. Second, the agency must have filed at least one completed cost report with the FI. Third, the agency must consistently demonstrate the ability to generate and maintain financial, statistical, and clinical information to support cost report and billing data. Fourth, and most important, the agency must be able to complete its M/C billing process in a timely manner. The Health Care Financing Administration (HCFA) considers timeliness to be when 85 percent of M/C visit services are billed within thirty days of being rendered.

## Settlement

Interim payments provide immediate financial resources for an agency, which must be reconciled by the FI at year's end. The mechanism to ensure payments are correct and to adjust for any differences is called *settlement.*

During the agency's FY, it may be noted that non-PIP or PIP payments are either overstated or understated as a result of the published M/C payment rate. To correct this error, the FI will perform a review of forecasted visit volume and the payment rate.

If adjustments are required during the current FY, the FI will take two actions to correct the situation. First, a corrected payment rate will be issued to non-PIP agencies. For PIP agencies, the biweekly check will be adjusted for the revised payment rate and visit volume.

Second, to correct for payments already made to the agency, the FI will issue a *retroactive settlement.* The retroactive settlement will either provide payment to or request payment from the agency to correct previous payments.

In principle, a *tentative settlement* is similar to a retroactive settlement, but the tentative is done after the close of the agency's FY and filing of the cost report. A cursory review of the cost report will indicate if payments to the agency were accurate. Any material differences will be corrected by the FI issuing a tentative settlement notice indicating if a payment is due the agency or the FI.

## Final Settlement

The last step in the reimbursement process is the final reconciliation of M/C reimbursable cost to interim payments. This is called the *final settlement.*

This calculation is performed after all agency billing and FI cost report audit review functions have been completed.

The final reimbursement is compared to interim, retroactive, and tentative payments made by the FI. The difference is reported in a *Notice of Provider Reimbursement* (NPR) letter. If payments were less than final reimbursement, a payment is sent by the FI to the agency. The opposite results in an overpayment situation; the agency sends a payment to the FI.

An unusual and unpleasant experience is when the FI calculates an overpayment and the agency is unable to make immediate payment. In this instance the agency can request an extended repayment schedule to extinguish the liability over an established period of time. On the surface this may seem simple. However, repayment schedule requirements imposed by the FI are known to be onerous and difficult. As previously mentioned, to avoid this situation it is important for the agency's financial department to monitor M/C payments and take appropriate action when indicated.

# BILLING FORMS

Billing requirements and supporting documentation of visit services are unique to home care and M/C. The actual bill is called the *UB-92* (UB stands for universal bill). Documentation of medical care is reported on the *HCFA-485, HCFA-486,* and *HCFA-487,* HCFA documentation.

The UB-92 contains a demographic description of

- the agency providing services
- the patient receiving services
- the patient's referring doctor
- medical diagnosis

Billing information indicates

- every home health service rendered
- the number of visits per service
- the charges for those services

The HCFA-485 is the *Home Health Plan of Treatment,* which is also known as plan of care, or physician's orders. The 485 specifies the illness and home care services required to treat the illness.

The HCFA-486 is the *End of Month Summary Form* that summarizes the first calendar month of patient progress. As of 1993, the 486 is no longer routinely submitted to the FI. In the event of an FI inquiry, the 486 is completed and submitted along with any other requested information.

The HCFA-487, or *Addendum,* is utilized for two purposes. First, the HCFA-485 and HCFA-486 may not contain enough space for detailed documentation, necessitating the addendum. Second, additions or changes to the plan of care must be ordered and signed for by a physician on a 487.

Information on HCFA forms can be found in Chapter 5.

# PROVIDER STATISTICAL AND REIMBURSEMENT SYSTEM

The billing of visits, charges associated with those visits, and the subsequent reimbursement by the FI need to be methodically recorded to determine interim and final settlement for M/C services rendered. The FIs instituted the *Provider Statistical and Reimbursement System* (PS&R) to handle the recording of such transactions.

The PS&R records the

- visit totals and charges
- approved reimbursement per visit
- detail of payments made to the agency under both non-PIP and PIP methodologies.

The FI utilizes the PS&R to report covered visits, approved charges, interim payments, and settlement adjustments on the final settlement cost report. It is important for the agency to carefully review PS&Rs from the FI. Any incorrect information should immediately be brought to the FI's attention before the final settlement is completed.

# GENERAL BILLING ISSUES

The first billing issue an agency faces is where to send the bills and supporting documentation. The answer is to the HCFA-designated FI.

Prior to 1986, the FI located geographically near an agency handled the processing and payment of bills and supporting documentation. In 1986, to streamline and make the process more efficient, HCFA established ten regional areas throughout the country. Discussion of FI functions will be addressed in Chapter 14.

The second issue facing an agency is how to submit the billing information to the FI. Currently, agencies are able to submit bills in one of two formats—*manual paper claims* or *electronic claims submission* (ECS).

The paper claim mode involves manually matching up the UB-92 with the appropriate HCFA documentation. After the match is made, the entire package is mailed to the FI.

The FI advocates utilization of a computer or electronic format because of cost inefficiencies associated with the manual process. Since HCFA has reduced funding to FIs for claims processing, FIs are stressing ECS for all home health agencies (HHAs).

With a capable management information system, an agency should be able to effectively utilize ECS. Submission may occur in any one of three formats—computer-to-computer via modem, electronic tape, or floppy disk.

Electronic claims submission offers an agency three advantages. First, agencies may receive their remittances back in an electronic media format. An agency with a system to accommodate electronic remittances will gain the advantage of having payments posted to their M/C receivable accounts automatically.

The second advantage is that electronic funds transfer to agencies on PIP. Agencies who submit bills and post payments electronically may have PIP reimbursement wired to their banks.

Third is miscellaneous expense savings associated with ECS. These savings occur through the elimination of postal costs and the reassignment of clerical staff who previously recorded, mailed, and posted M/C claims.

## Statute of Limitation

The last issue an agency should be cognizant of is the statute of limitations for submitting M/C claims. Statute stipulates that claims for the first nine months of the year have to be submitted by the end of the subsequent year. The final three months of billing have to be submitted by the end of the second subsequent year.

The following example should clear up confusion. An agency provides visits from January 1, 1995, through December 31, 1995. Billing claims for the period January 1, 1995, through September 30, 1995, must be submitted to the FI by *December 31, 1996.* Claims from October 1, 1995, through December 31, 1995, have until *December 31, 1997* to be submitted.

Claims not submitted by the agency to the FI within the statute will be rejected for payment. Exceptions to the statute will only be made in the event of extraordinary circumstances. Such a circumstance would be loss of claims, accompanied by supporting documentation from a private mail delivery service.

# CONCLUSION

Timely payment for visits and services rendered is one of the most important financial issues an agency is faced with. Without a predictable and acceptable cash flow, day-to-day routine operations can be temporarily, or in extreme cases permanently, damaged.

Monitoring of the payment rate is required to assure reimbursement will not result in any overpayments or underpayments by the FI. Timely billing of visit services is necessary to guarantee prompt payment.

## *Suggested Readings*

U.S. Department of Health and Human Services Health Care Financing Administration. (1994). *Medicare Provider Reimbursement Manual HCFA–Pub 15–1*. Chapters 24 and 29.

U.S. Department of Health and Human Services Health Care Financing Administration. *Medicare Home Health Agency Manual, HCFA–Pub 11*. Chapters 2 and 4.

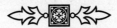

# CHAPTER

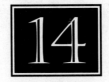

# Other Medicare Issues

Timothy Riordan

Previous chapters have focused on the Medicare (M/C) situations of a singular free-standing or hospital-based agency. In this chapter, broader treatment of the M/C reimbursement environment will include *fiscal intermediaries, home health agency (HHA) chain organizations,* and the concept of *related organizations.*

# FISCAL INTERMEDIARIES

The establishment of M/C as a health care payer in 1966 posed operational questions and issues for the federal government.

- How was the program to be administered?
- Who would make payments for services rendered?
- How will the *Health Care Financing Administration* (HCFA) make payments to the vast number of health care organizations and providers of services?
- How will HCFA know if payments made for services are proper and reasonable?
- What mechanism is in place to ensure against fraud and abuse?

To answer these and other questions, HCFA established regional fiscal intermediaries (FI). The FI would ostensibly be a liaison between the federal government and health care organizations providing care and service to M/C beneficiaries. Health care organizations, or *providers,* include hospitals, skilled nursing facilities, HHAs, and outpatient rehabilitation clinics.

The primary function of the FI is to make payment for services provided. The FI also takes steps to ensure the appropriateness of payments through audit and review functions.

The establishment of payments for HHA services starts with the FI promulgating a reimbursement rate at the start of the agency's fiscal year (FY). Please refer to Chapter 13 for detailed information.

The initial payment rate needs to be as accurate as possible. The FI is as concerned as the agency in avoiding material overpayments and underpayments for services. The information utilized to calculate an initial rate is taken from the most recent audited or *as submitted* cost report data. Then the FI begins a sequential process.

## Desk Audit

After the FI receives the cost report, questionnaires, financial statements, and all other required material from the agency, a *desk audit* review is performed. This review is guided by a desk audit program that details the procedures to be followed.

A desk audit review is an analysis for completeness and accuracy of the cost report and all other submitted material. Questionnaires and financial statements are reviewed for reimbursement issues. Also, a review of material on file for prior years is conducted to identify problems that may affect the current year.

After the desk audit, the FI will update the reimbursement rate in effect. If the desk audit calculates a rate that is materially different than the initial rate, the revised rate will be established. This may result in a tentative settlement where previous payments made to the agency are adjusted. The FI may consider completing a final settlement of the cost report if the amount of M/C reimbursement involved is insignificant or if prior years' review found no problems with the cost report submission.

A desk audit review may trigger further review if reimbursement or prior year problems are identified. If further review is found to be necessary, it takes the form of a *no-audit* or *field audit*.

### No-Audit

A no-audit results from a desk audit review that notes minor problems. A request for supporting schedules or other information will be made to resolve any questions. The no-audit may be conducted for one to three days at the FI's office or on-site at the agency.

### Field Audit

A field audit is a comprehensive review of the submitted cost report. It will take place at the agency for the purpose of readily obtaining supporting documentation.

As with a desk audit, the auditors conducting the field review follow a program. The program is dictated by the results of the desk audit. These results may necessitate a *full audit* or *limited audit scope program*.

### Full Audit

A full scope audit program calls for a review of all cost and statistical supporting documentation. Review of agency financial policies and procedures will establish a comfort level for the FI that financial data reported is correct.

### Limited Scope Audit

In between a no-audit and a full scope audit is a limited scope audit. This audit addresses specific items noted in the desk audit review, the current handling of prior year adjustments, or other reimbursement issues.

## On-Site Audit Process

Both full and limited scope audits begin with written notice that an audit is scheduled. The notification requests that supporting cost report documentation and other items are ready for the auditors on their arrival.

At an *entrance conference,* the auditors meet with agency management for introductory purposes and to discuss the nature of the audit. During the audit, the auditors may find reimbursement issues that require adjustments. These adjustments are discussed and resolved with agency management either at the time they are found or at the close of the audit. After the auditors have completed their activities, an *exit conference* is held. The auditors discuss their findings and adjustments with agency management. The agency then has the right to verbally rebut any of the auditors' findings. If the agency can successfully defend itself against a proposed audit adjustment, the FI will not make the adjustment during the final settlement process.

Within thirty days of the exit conference, the FI sends an *audit report notice* to the agency detailing all proposed adjustments to be made to the cost report. Also included with the notice is a *management letter* detailing financial or other policy and procedure deficiencies.

In order for the agency to preserve its right to appeal, it must respond in writing within thirty days of the audit report notice. If deficiencies are mentioned in the management letter, the agency is expected to take corrective action for subsequent cost reporting time periods.

After mailing audit adjustments applicable to the submitted cost report, the FI will calculate a final settlement. The final settlement is composed of the following

- *Notice of Provider Reimbursement* (NPR) letter detailing the final M/C reimbursable cost and the final settlement payment due either the agency or the FI
- audit report, including the management letter, that was previously sent to the agency
- cost report revised for audit adjustments
- notification of final M/C payment rate

### *The Notice of Provider Reimbursement Letter*

The NPR letter has two date-sensitive items that must be addressed by the agency. First, if an overpayment has occurred, payment is to be made by the agency to the FI within thirty days. If the payment is not made by the required date, the FI may either impose interest on the payment or may recoup the amount by reducing interim payments. Conversely, payments determined to be due the agency will be made within thirty days of the dated NPR letter.

Second, any items to be appealed for the cost report year must be submitted within 180 days after receipt of the NPR letter. Such items include the disputing of an audit adjustment or other items affecting the calculation of M/C reimbursement on the cost report.

Agencies that are over the M/C caps may utilize the appeal process to obtain relief from the caps for unique expenses incurred.

For example, a provider may incur additional expense for providing additional security for nurses working in high crime areas. If the agency feels the costs applicable to security are unique to the agency and not addressed in the promulgation of the caps, the agency may appeal to have those costs reimbursed.

# HOME HEALTH AGENCY CHAIN ORGANIZATIONS

The financial and reimbursement topics covered thus far have had a single HHA as its focus. However, there are home care organizations that have multiple HHA sites.

Proprietary and not-for-profit HHAs with multiple sites are known as *chain organizations,* or *chains.* The one defining characteristic of a chain is that all sites are controlled by a single organization.

Chains are usually organized with *site offices* and a *corporate* or *home office.* Site offices are located throughout the region served by the chain. Visits and other clinical services are provided from the sites.

The home office is where management, financial, computer, billing, and other administrative functions for all sites occur. Clinical services do not originate from the home office. Chains consider the centralization of common functions to be efficient.

Site offices are considered discrete providers by M/C. Their individual direct and overhead expenses are reimbursed by M/C through the mechanisms previously explained in Chapter 12.

Since the home office is not a provider of clinical services, M/C will not reimburse the home office directly for expenses incurred for providing services to the individual sites. Reimbursement occurs indirectly on the individual site's cost reports.

The mechanism for reimbursing home office costs begins with the home office completing its own cost report. After expense is reported and classified, an allocation of expense to the individual sites is then stepped down. Only home office expense related to the home care services provided by the sites are to be allocated to the sites. All other expense related to other types of businesses will not be allocated to the site for reimbursement under M/C.

The home office cost report utilizes three types of expense allocation methodologies—*direct, functional,* and *pooled.*

## Direct Allocation of Expense

The allocation process first requires that any costs that can be identified with a particular site be directly allocated to that site. For example, if the home office incurred consulting expense related to a problem or concern of site A, the expense will be directly allocated to site A.

## Functional Allocation of Expense

The next step requires the identification of expenses that can be functionally allocated to the sites. The basis for functional allocation must be equitable for purposes of ensuring the individual sites receive the proper amount of expense. For instance, expenses incurred for the payroll department for the entire chain are reported on the home office cost report. An acceptable basis for allocating payroll department expense to each site is basing it on payroll checks issued per site. If site A has twice as many employees and paychecks issued than site B, site A will receive twice as much payroll department expense during the allocation process.

## Pooled Allocation of Expense

After the direct and functional costs are allocated, the remaining home office costs are to be allocated under pooled cost methodology. This methodology is similar to the allocation of administrative and general (A&G) expense on the HHA cost report. Expenses that are difficult to allocate, such as home office utility expense, will be stepped down to the sites using the direct expense at each site and the accumulated cost allocation process described in Chapter 12.

### Reporting of Allocated Expense

After all expense is allocated to the sites, it is reported on the site cost report as an A&G expense and is subject to the same reimbursement principles as all other site A&G expense. It should be noted, as with all other reimbursable expense, the home office allocation will be reviewed by the FI for reasonableness and appropriateness.

## Single Intermediary Designation

A chain organization with sites in different states may have to deal with multiple FIs. This may be problematic since FIs may differ in how they handle M/C reimbursement issues. To accommodate the varying interpretations, one chain may have a variety of operational and financial policies and procedures to accommodate each FI's requirements.

To standardize, and hopefully avoid confusion, a chain may apply to HCFA for a single intermediary designation. One FI is appointed to handle the billing, cost report submission and audit, appeal, and other reimbursement functions for the entire chain. Such a designation allows the home office and the sites to become familiar with the idiosyncrasies of one intermediary.

# RELATED ORGANIZATIONS

Compared to a traditional M/C certified agency, a home care program may provide more, or different, services. Indeed, many agencies have other programs or *related organizations.*

The definition of a related organization is a program or organization that is associated with, affiliated with, or controlled by the agency. The agency usually provides administrative and financial services in a manner similar to a home office in a chain organization.

Examples of related organizations include HHA-based hospice programs, private duty nursing organizations, or individual states that may have alternative home care programs that do not provide M/C certified services. Therefore the agency may treat these types of programs as related organizations of the certified agency.

In performing the M/C cost report audit, the FI will review any related organizations and how their relationship impacts the agency's reimbursable expense. Any expense that is allocated through such a relationship will be reviewed for reasonableness and appropriateness. For example, if any of the agency's A&G expense is entirely for the operation of a related organization, the FI will not allow that expense to be included with M/C reimbursable expense.

## CONCLUSION

The M/C environment is not confined to the single certified agency. Other organizations, both federal and private, interact with the certified to provide funding for patient care services. The certified itself may have, or belong to, other organizations.

The function and purpose of the FI is to provide and ensure the accuracy of payments for services rendered to M/C beneficiaries. Chains and related organizations offer centralized administrative services and enable certified programs to utilize additional resources efficiently in the provision of services.

### *Suggested Reading*

U.S. Department of Health and Human Services Health Care Financing Administration. (1994). *Medicare Provider Reimbursement Manual HCFA-Pub 15–1.* Chapters 10, 21, and 29.

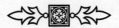

# CHAPTER

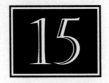

15

# The Budget Process

**Timothy Riordan**

The importance of planning future financial operations, or *budgeting,* cannot be stressed enough. Currently there is greater demand on agency resources to provide visits and other services to patients in an environment of constricting payments by third-party payers.

As a result, agencies are well-advised to budget with the following in mind.

• What are the estimated types and volume of services for the upcoming time period?
• What will be the expenses applicable to forecasted services?
• What revenues can be expected from forecasted services?

Once a draft budget has been prepared, the agency can estimate its financial future for the upcoming period. Potential financial problems can be identified and hopefully resolved by the time the budget is accepted. A reasonable and responsible budget will allow an agency to do what it does best—provide quality services in a cost-efficient manner to its patients.

## THE BUDGET PROCESS

The first step in the budget process is to define the *budget mission statement.* This statement is a summary of agency goals (overall mission statement) and the financial techniques for achieving and sustaining the goals.

Defining the statement necessitates participation of clinical, administrative, and financial staff. Input from these areas helps assure the statement is in balance from a clinical and financial perspective. Additionally, the long-term strategies to accomplish the mission should have been developed with, and by, the appropriate divisions.

Once the budget mission statement is complete, a *budget timetable* has to be established. The actual budget time frame depends on the agency itself. Most begin the process four months before the start of the fiscal year (FY). For example, if the FY begins July 1, then the budget process begins March 1. This allows for adequate preparation, review, and approval of the budget by the start of the FY. The timetable should specify

• date when submission of forecast information from all agency departments must be accomplished. The patient care section needs to forecast the types and volume of services to be provided; payroll will submit salary and merit raise material; accounts payable provides nonsalary expense information, and general accounting will supply all other required financial information.
• when the budget department will review submitted information and assemble a draft of the budget
• date when the draft budget will be reviewed by senior management for appropriateness and reasonableness. It is expected that financial and clinical operations will "break even" or show a modest surplus for the upcoming time period.
• when the budget will then be presented to the agency's Board of Directors for review and, hopefully, approval

The board-approved budget should be shared with all agency management to provide a sense of fiscal direction. The sharing of fiscal and budgetary information will make managers aware of overall goals and their responsibilities in achieving them.

# VOLUME ESTIMATE

The first step in budget development is the determination of expected volume of services to be provided in the coming FY. Visit and hour volumes for both *professional* and *paraprofessional* services need to be estimated.

## Visits

Professional service disciplines include skilled nursing (SN), physical therapy (PT), occupational therapy (OT), speech pathology (SP), and medical social work (MSW). The unit of measure for professional services is *visits*.

Due to staffing shortages in recent times, the calculation of professional visit volume should begin with the availability of direct care staff. Direct care staff, also known as field staff, consists of employees of the agency and is counted in units known as *full-time equivalents* (FTEs).

An FTE is a set number of hours worked during one year. If an agency requires an individual to work from 8:30 A.M. to 5:30 P.M. daily, five days per week, then the FTE is 2,080 hours per year (9 hours per day less one hour for meal multiplied by 5 days per week multiplied by 52 weeks per year). The amount of hours varies with the work schedules required by the agencies.

Determination of how many visits each FTE of direct care staff can provide on a daily and annual basis is the next step in the budget process. The annual number of expected visits should account for lost days to vacation, holiday, sick time, and any other unique, paid nonproductive time.

Productivity of direct care staff is specific to each agency's patient situation. For example, an agency located in an urban area with patients grouped closely together should have a higher daily productivity compared to a rural agency where the distance between patients is greater. The following daily productivity visit ranges may prove useful in budgeting: nursing, 4–7; therapies, 4–6; and medical social service, 3–4.

In calculating visit volume, a distinction has to be made between visits that are *billable* and *nonbillable*. Although both types have applicable expenses, only billable visits will be utilized for calculating revenue. Nonbillables consist of supervisory, assessment, or other *nonrevenue generating* visits, and may be considered simply an overhead expense.

Upon determining clinical productivity per FTE and the number of available FTEs, multiplying one by the other will equal annual visits. If a nursing FTE can produce 1,300 visits per year and an agency has 20 nursing FTEs, the budget volume would be 26,000 nursing visits (1,300 visits per nurse multiplied by 20 nurses).

The calculation of HHA visits and hours may be linked with the provision of nursing visits. Using the above example, historical data might indicate that for every nursing visit provided, 2 HHA visits are provided. Therefore the agency can budget 52,000 HHA visits (26,000 nursing visits multiplied by 2 HHA visits per nursing visit).

## Hours

The main paraprofessional service provided by agencies is home health aide (HHA). Given the nature of HHA services, the units of measure are both visits and *hours*.

The estimate of hours is critical as hours vary for each payer. Medicare (M/C) beneficiaries can receive four hours of service on every HHA visit for a usual total of twenty hours per week. Other payers reimbursing for custodial care services may require eight, twelve, or even twenty-four hours of care on every visit. Given disparities, estimating hours will allow for accurate revenue and expense. Historical HHA visit and hours data for budgeting is a helpful guideline for this part of budget preparation.

After determining HHA visit volume, the applicable hours must be budgeted. Again, historical data will provide average hours per visit ratios for the different payers from which an agency receives reimbursement. Multiplying the ratios by the number of visits in each payer will provide budgeted HHA hours. If historical data reports 4 hours as the average number per M/C HHA visit and the agency will provide 30,000 M/C HHA visits, budgeted M/C hours will be 120,000 (4 hours per visit multiplied by 30,000 visits).

## Other Utilization

The next component of the volume calculation is to determine the visits that will be made through overtime (OT) or by contract. Visits to be made through overtime can again be estimated by utilizing historical data. Assuming 1,500 hours were paid in OT, the actual number of hours *worked* was 1,000 (1,000 multiplied by time and one-half equals 1,500 *paid* OT hours). As a professional visit is expected to approximate 1 hour, then there will be 1,000 OT visits made.

Contract visits are estimated by determining where staffing deficiencies require utilization of contractors to cover visits. Contractor availability must be acknowledged and placed in perspective in relation to achievable visit volume.

Overtime and contractor expense is useful in justifying the need for additional staff. For instance, if there were 1,000 OT visits and 1,600 contractor visits, that is the equivalent of 2 FTEs if the expected annual visits per FTE is 1,300.

# SALARY EXPENSE

The most significant expense item in a budget is salary or wages. Since employees, as defined by the Internal Revenue Service (IRS), provide the majority of visits for an agency, it is important to remember that visits and salary expense are dependant on each other.

First, FTEs have to be determined for both direct care staff and administrative and support staff. Since the budgeted visit volume for services provided by employees has been established, the number of direct field staff is already known.

After direct care staff, all other FTEs come from case managers and coordinators, administration, supervisory, finance, management information systems, clerical, and other support service areas. Adjustments, both increases and decreases, may be necessary to support staff FTEs to compensate for changes in visit volume.

## Assigning Salary Dollars

Once total agency FTEs are budgeted, salaries are assigned. Salary information can be obtained from the human resources or payroll departments. Additionally, these departments provide the approved merit pool increases for the upcoming year.

Upon completion of the basic salary expense, additional factors such as OT, temporary employees, coverage for vacations, and other absences are considered. Historical experience should serve as a guide for the budgeting of these expenses.

# OTHER THAN SALARY EXPENSE

After salary expense has been accounted for, all other expense associated with providing services must be recognized. The major types of expense and common methodologies used in budget preparation follow.

## Fringe Benefits

Directly associated with salaries are *fringe benefits* expense. Fringe benefits may be budgeted by estimating the amount of payroll taxes, pension expense, health insurance, and other benefits applicable to budgeted salaries. Once this amount is known, it may be expressed as a percentage of salaries. Therefore if budgeted salary expense are revised, fringes may be easily recalculated.

For example, if fringe benefits are estimated to be $1 million on salaries of $5 million, the 20 percent ($1 million divided by $5 million) figure can be used for revision purposes. If salaries increase to $6 million, fringe benefits would increase to $1.2 million ($6 million multiplied by 20 percent).

## Professional and Paraprofessional Contract Expense

Expense for contracted clinical services is a major expense item for an agency that does not provide the service directly. Once expected contract visits and hours are calculated, the utilization may be multiplied by the budgeted rate for such services.

In the following example, an agency provides all HHA services through vendors. Approximately 200,000 hours will be rendered in the FY and the agency has negotiated to pay $12 per hour. Total FY budget contract expense will be $2.4 million (200,000 hours multiplied by $12 per hour).

## Property, Plant, and Equipment Expense

Plant and equipment owned by the agency is depreciated annually. The general accounting department can provide budget depreciation expense by utilizing ledgers that summarize asset information. For rented plant and equipment, the rental agreements will provide the rent expense for the upcoming year.

## Home Medical Equipment and Medical Supplies

Expense applicable to home medical equipment (HME) and medical supplies is difficult to accurately budget. This is due to shifts in average patient acuity or diagnosis from one FY to another.

An example illustrates the difficulty. If the historical HME and supplies expense is $50 per patient, the budget expense is calculated by multiplying the amount by the annual patient count. However, the actual year may find a more acute patient population requiring an average of $100 in expense. This will result in actual expense materially exceeding its budget.

Historical data is a starting point in budgeting for HME and supplies expense. To allow for any uncertainties, a contingency amount may be also included in the budget.

## Office Supplies

Routine business supplies are budgeted by using the most current expense data available. These expenses are then *trended forward* to the budget year. Trended forward is taking a current expense and multiplying it by an inflation factor to determine its future worth. Other reasonable estimates can be made if there is confidence in the methods used.

# REVENUE

The first step in calculating revenue is to determine the payer mix of the patients who are to receive services. Current third-party activity, historical information, and demographic changes can provide good indicators of payer mix.

For instance, prior year utilization indicated M/C was 65 percent of total visits rendered. Current assessment of the patient population indicates the M/C population is expected to grow. The budget payer mix would have M/C at 70 percent of visits to be rendered.

Visits and hours may then be assigned by payer mix and service. Calculated visits and hours for both professional and paraprofessional services are then assigned third-party reimbursement rates.

## Retrospective Reimbursement

The determination of M/C and other cost-based retrospective rates should follow the respective cost-reporting guidelines. A projected cost report utilizing previously budgeted volume and expense needs to be completed in order to determine the cost per visit to be reimbursed. The cost per visit is then compared to the cost per visit limitations, or *caps,* promulgated by the payer for the coming year. Either the cost per visit or cap, whichever is lower, should be assigned to the anticipated payer visit volume.

## Prospective Reimbursement

Third-party prospective reimbursement rates already provide the *base year* rates in accordance with predefined regulations. Base year is a time period established by a payer from which future years are trended forward. The budget process in this situation is to estimate how to trend the base year rate forward to the budget year. Hopefully the third-party insurer is able to provide advance notice of the trend factor. If not, the agency has to do its best to utilize the most current published economic information available and determine an appropriate trend factor. The base year rate multiplied by the estimated trend factor will provide the budgeted rate to be assigned to the applicable utilization.

## Revenue Calculation and Bad Debt

After determining reimbursement rates for each payer and discipline, the rates are multiplied by the appropriate utilization to determine total revenue for the coming year. The next step is to determine how much of that revenue is collectible.

Utilizing revenue collection data from prior years will enable an agency to budget the *bad debt* portion of revenue. Bad debt is that portion of revenue unlikely to be collected. From this data, bad debt percentages can be estimated and multiplied against total revenue to calculate bad debt. The total revenue less bad debt will give budgeted *net revenue.*

# CONCLUSION

At this point the agency should have all the components in place to forecast the upcoming year. Concise and detailed pictures of the upcoming year may be presented to the agency's Board of Directors in two formats—the budgeted profit and loss statement, and the cost report.

Once the board-approved budget is complete and the upcoming year commences, the agency has a valuable tool to monitor fiscal progress. The budget can be compared to monthly fiscal results to highlight material variances. Material variances reviewed by agency management can be utilized to identify operational or other fiscal problems as early as possible. Once these problems are identified, the agency can take steps to resolve them.

The budget process for agencies is not well-documented in the home care industry. Indeed, the processes are usually unique to every agency. The uniqueness of each agency leads to different sets of financial circumstances and, accordingly, customization of the budgeting process. The process in this chapter reflects the author's own experience in budgeting.

# CHAPTER

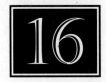

16

# Current and Future Financial Issues

**Timothy Riordan**

The nation's recent concern for health care reform, and the Clinton Administration's mission of reform, has caused individual agencies and the home care industry as a whole to re-think their purpose and future. Health care reform, along with the Health Care Financing Administration's (HCFA) movement from a retrospective to a prospective or other type of payment system, signals the advent of a new financial era for home care. This chapter will focus on current and future financial issues.

# FEDERAL REIMBURSEMENT REDUCTIONS

A reduction of payments for home care occurred in the fall of 1993 with the passage of President Clinton's *Omnibus Reconciliation Act of 1993* (OBRA-93). The act reduced home care expenditures in two ways.

First, Medicare (M/C) *routine cost limitations,* or caps, for services of cost report years beginning July 1, 1993, are frozen for the two subsequent time periods. If an agency has a fiscal year (FY) of January 1, 1994, through December 31, 1994, the 1994 caps will remain the same for 1995 and 1996. Those agencies consistently over the caps will not receive any increase in their M/C reimbursement rate until 1997.

Second, the *administrative and general* (A&G) add-on to the caps for hospital-based home health agencies was eliminated. Previous to OBRA-93, HCFA recognized that hospital-based agencies had additional overhead expense from the sponsoring hospital through the step-down process. To reimburse for the expense, HCFA allowed an A&G add-on, which resulted in an additional 12 to 15 percent to the reimbursement per visit. The elimination will have an especially adverse financial impact on those agencies over the caps.

## Co-payments

OBRA-93 is just the beginning of federal cost-cutting. Other federal proposals would institute co-payments for M/C home care services. Co-payment is the portion of a medical service charge for which the beneficiary is responsible. If a payer has a 20 percent co-payment on a skilled nursing visit charge of $100, then the beneficiary is responsible for $20 ($100 multiplied by 20 percent) of the charge. Different proposals have M/C beneficiaries paying anywhere from 10 to 20 percent of charges. Those opposing co-payments lead to the argument that overhead expense will increase, since the likelihood of collecting from the patient is poor at best. In addition, some argue it will restrict the provision of services since they believe M/C beneficiaries faced with co-payments may forgo services to avoid the expense.

# STATE REIMBURSEMENT REDUCTIONS

Payment constriction is occurring on the state level as well. Increasingly, Medicaid (M/A) programs are implementing reimbursement rate freezes, or reductions, to balance state budgets.

For instance, New York State M/A has implemented various forms of reimbursement reductions. Aside from an overall cap for reimbursement rates, there is a cap to particular A&G expense. Those agencies with A&G expense in excess of 28 percent of total expense have had their reimbursement rate adjusted to eliminate the excess. Another reimbursement reduction was the implementation of a *cash receipts assessment.* This assessment, similar if not identical to a tax, requires certified home health agencies (HHAs) to remit 0.60 percent of all cash receipts back to the state.

There are various payers who, due to financial circumstances, find it necessary to reduce payments for home care services. In a shrinking reimbursement environment, agencies are looking to cut expenses, provide services in a more efficient manner, open new markets, and find business opportunities.

# PROSPECTIVE PAYMENT

Subject to regulatory limitations, the current M/C system allows for payment of home care services through a retrospective cost-based system. This means the source of M/C reimbursement is expenses incurred for the actual provision of services to M/C beneficiaries.

Critics of retrospective payment contend there is no incentive for HHAs to be cost-efficient in the delivery of patient services. Those agencies with a M/C cost per visit rate below the *routine cost limitations,* or caps, may find it to their advantage to incur more expense, which can then be reimbursed up to the caps.

The critics believe a *prospective payment system* (PPS) is the way to reduce M/C costs. The concept of PPS was developed in the early 1980s for M/C payments to hospitals. The Reagan Administration, concerned with spiraling hospital costs, sought to limit or contain M/C reimbursement for those services.

Prospective payment was the impetus for *Diagnostic Related Groups* (DRGs). Each DRG has an assigned, single, preset payment for the in-hospital treatment of that illness.

Hospitals able to provide efficient care benefit since their costs are below the DRG reimbursement and any savings are retained by the hospital. Hospitals providing care at costs greater than DRG payments will find expense outpacing revenue, which may lead to a myriad of financial problems, not the least of which is insolvency.

The Omnibus Reconciliation Act of 1987 (OBRA-87) and of 1990 (OBRA-90) mandated HCFA to undertake a project to develop, test, and evaluate various methodologies of reimbursing home care services on a prospective basis. Prospective payment, in all likelihood, will be affected in two stages.

## Individual Payment Rates and Disaggregation

The first phase of prospective payment for home care was completed in the fall of 1994. In this phase each of the six individual home care disciplines was assigned an individual payment rate. Therefore no matter what the cost of a visit for a specific discipline, the payment amount is already assigned by HCFA for that discipline.

This is similar to the M/C, or caps promulgated in 1985. The application of the caps forbade the offsetting of expense over the caps in one discipline by other disciplines below the caps. This application was known as *disaggregation.* Vigorous protest from the home care industry resulted in its repeal in the following year.

The first phase process of assigning individual discipline rates was predicated on a *budget or cost neutral* outcome. In other words, transforming from retrospective fee for service payment environment to a prospective system would not result in any additional monetary outlays by the M/C program. To be budget neutral, it was determined the individual payment rates would have to be set at approximately 83 percent of the M/C caps.

As with the implementation of DRGs for hospitals, the outcome of the first phase will benefit those HHAs that are already comfortably under the caps. Those agencies above the caps will need to be more efficient and reduce costs in order to survive.

## Per Episode

The second phase will be a *per episode* payment methodology, which is very similar to hospital DRG payments. Home care services provided to M/C beneficiaries with a specific illness, such as congestive heart failure, will have a predetermined payment assigned by HCFA. No matter how many visits are provided to a patient with a diagnosis of congestive heart failure, the M/C payment will be the set amount for the particular episode.

## Bundling

A proposed alternative to home care PPS is *bundling.* Bundling involves increasing the hospital DRG payment to include payment for post–acute services, including home care. The hospital would be responsible to reimburse home care agencies and other non-hospital providers for services rendered to patients.

Although HCFA is required to report on the home care PPS project in the near future, it is believed the implementation of such a complex system will take significant time. However, proponents continue to advocate for PPS, believing it offers incentives to operate in a cost-effective manner. Those incentives are absent in the retrospective system. They also argue it will simplify and make more predictable the M/C reimbursement of expenses.

# CHARITY CARE

*Charity care,* or *free care,* is the provision of home care service at a reduced charge or at no charge. The reduction or elimination of the agency's published charge occurs when a preadmission financial assessment finds only partial or no payment will be realized from the patient.

Certain states or localities mandate the provision of charity care. For example, in New York State there are established minimum charity care provisions for various kinds of agencies. Voluntary agencies must provide an amount equal to or greater than 2.00 percent of certified total operating costs. Public agencies are required to provide 3.33 percent or more in charity care. The patient can not have any third-party payment source, and must have a household income less than 200 percent of the federal poverty level to qualify for charity care.

# MANAGED CARE

People in the 1990s are witnessing a revolution in the way health care is paid for and delivered. Two concerns are driving the change. First is the belief that health care is a right and privilege, and that all Americans should have some access to care. Second, the cost of care is out of sync with the rest of the economy. Elected government officials, private businesses, and the public are now in the forefront of the health care reform movement.

The threat of reform has led to the advent of more widespread *managed care.* Managed care is the purchase of health care services, which focus on the utilization and the price paid for those services. Private businesses are considered the prime payers through premiums paid for health care services; their employees are considered the consumers of such services. Business philosophy regarding the purchase of coverage is now similar to that of all other purchases—get the best possible services at the lowest possible prices. As a result of this evolving philosophy, different types of health care organizations have developed. *Health maintenance organizations* (HMOs), *preferred provider organizations* (PPOs), and *physician—hospital organizations* (PHOs) are offering services to businesses, usually at *discounted prices.*

Given the current environment and the certainty of future changes, HHAs must conduct strategic planning to ensure their place in the "new world." Agencies will no longer receive the majority of patient referrals through traditional processes. They will have to attract customers by aligning themselves with one or more of the previously mentioned organizations and networks.

# LONG-TERM STRATEGY

The financial segment of an agency's long-term strategy should be determining at what price services can be provided. Pricing strategy may be the traditional *cost per visit or hour, cost per episode,* a *capitated rate,* or a combination of these, depending on the payer.

## Cost Per Visit or Hour and Episode

The cost per visit or hour is easily determined from the M/C cost report. As mentioned in Chapter 12, the cost report should be prepared on an interim basis and has to be filed with the M/C fiscal intermediary (FI) annually. An agency negotiating managed care reimbursement rates may use a current cost report as a baseline for pricing and discounting services.

Pricing agency services on a per episode basis requires two components for *every* type of illness or diagnosis an agency treats. First, cost per visit or hour information is needed as described above. Second, clinical data detailing the type and number of services *per* diagnosis is needed. An agency needs to access, from its management information system, all diagnoses the agency has treated, the professional and paraprofessional services utilized in the treatment of each diagnosis, the number of visits by individual discipline, and the visit aggregate.

From this information the agency can determine the average consumption of services per diagnosis. These services multiplied by the cost per visit or hour will determine the average cost per episode. Again, the agency may use such averages in negotiating payment rates.

## Capitation

Capitation is the latest developing reimbursement mechanisms for home care services. Although already in place for inpatient and outpatient hospital services, the home care industry is in its infancy for capitation reimbursement.

The basis of capitation is that a third-party payer wants to purchase health care services for its members in advance. The payer contacts health care providers, states the services required, and asks for a *price*. The price is in the form of *X* dollars per member over a stated period of time.

In order to respond to a request, the provider must evaluate important aspects of the population to be covered. First, can it develop a price, or capitated rate, that enables the provision of required services? Second, what effect, if any, will there be on the quality of services? Third, will a negative response result in a loss of patient referrals?

The development of a capitated rate for home care services is difficult if the home care needs of the *capitated lives* are unknown or understated. Similar to the funding of pensions for the future of retirees, an agency must have actuarial information on the expected amount of home care services to be rendered. The actuaries will study a catchment area, utilizing available health care data, census, and other information. From their studies a determination of *expected* home care services required for the population can be estimated.

### Case Study

Payer A insures the health service needs of 100,000 members. To provide home care services to its members, it requests that Agency B submit a capitated payment rate for review.

From preparing cost reports, Agency B knows the average cost of home care services per patient is $400. From actuarial studies performed on the population of its catchment area, it has determined for every 100,000 individuals, 500 will require home health services.

The total cost of services expected to be provided for Payer A's 100,000 members is $200,000 ($400 per patient multiplied by 500 patients). The annual capitated rate per member is $2 ($200,000 expected cost of services divided by 100,000 members).

Capitation is a reimbursement system with mixed blessings. The agency is guaranteed a fixed stream of patient service revenue from the third-party payer. However, the development of the capitated rate is difficult, and may be easily outdated if there is a significant change in the health care needs of the population receiving service. Should this happen, the agency may have competing needs—balancing the costs and being able to provide quality services. It would be beneficial for agencies to negotiate a *stop loss clause* in the agreement to limit financial liabilities.

As the capitated reimbursement methodology evolves, certain hybrid systems will be offered to agencies. One such hybrid is *active patient* capitation. Active patient is tailored for sick beneficiaries with specific diagnoses. Fees that are higher than normal capitated rates are paid for beneficiaries who access services from the provider. Although the fees are higher and the patient population is not large, there are high costs associated with the care provided. Thus the opportunity for higher profits under active capitation comes with the risk of great losses.

## CONCLUSION

The home care industry is facing a challenging and interesting period in its history. Agencies will continue to provide basic and customary services, but the form of reimbursement will change, as will the breadth of services.

Financial case management will lead the way in containing the cost of services by limiting and negotiating reimbursement to agencies. Reimbursement will move to a prospective per episode or capitated basis, not the traditional, soon to be historical, retrospective cost per visit methodology.

## *Suggested Readings*

Hogue, E. E. (1993). Negotiating discount agreements for managed care contracts. *Hospital Home Health* 10:8:122–24.

Hoyer, B. (1994). The anatomy of PPS: Part 1 of a series. *National Association for Home Care Report, 582,* 1–4.

Lutz, S. (1993). Hospitals continue move into home care. *Modern Health Care, 23*(4), 28–30, 32.

Waldrop, S. (1995). With "active patient" capitation you could score profits on even the most expensive patients. . . . *home health line, 20*(2), 3–4.

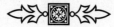

# PART THREE

---

## DELIVERY OF PATIENT SERVICES

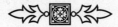

# CHAPTER

# Recruitment

**Stephanie Taylor Davis**

In order to establish and maintain an effective home health agency (HHA), consideration must be given to the categories of staff needed to provide patients with appropriate care. Compliance with state and federal regulations and professional standards are equally important components of the recruitment process.

# DEFINITIONS AND TYPES OF STAFF

In order to be considered a "full service" agency under the Medicare (M/C) conditions of participation (COPs), an agency must directly provide at least 67 percent of one of the qualifying services (skilled nursing, physical therapy (PT) or speech therapy). Other M/C reimbursed services include occupational therapy (OT), medical social work (MSW), and personal care (home health aides [HHAs]). Depending on individual state or local regulations, agencies with a long-term component may require additional professional personnel such as audiologists and nutritionists.

## Employees Versus Contractors

Employees, according to Internal Revenue Service (IRS) guidelines, are individuals whose primary source of income originates in one organization that has a responsibility to withhold taxes from wages earned. An agency may hire staff who are either full-time, part-time, or per visit (also known as fee for service, or per diem), in any combination needed to meet patient care requirements. Independent contractors, who qualify as such by IRS definition, are *not* employees of the agency. Independent contractors can be corporations or entities such as licensed agencies, and may supply some or all of a *non-qualifying* service such as personal care workers.

## Groups of Staff

Within the agency there are well-defined groups of staff. *Direct care staff,* or field staff, are those professionals and paraprofessionals who have physical contact with the patient and/or family. *Administrative staff* have managerial responsibility for the coordination and direction of a discrete or multifaceted group of staff. These managers may or may not have contact with patients or families; if they do have contact it will be limited in most instances. *Support staff* are the personnel who provide support to the field staff such as escorts/drivers, medical records clerks, clinical secretaries, and so forth.

### Direct Field Staff

*Registered nurses (RNs),* are what M/C defines as the *skilled nursing* component of home care. The qualifications for an RN are not universally delineated. However, if a common sense approach is used, new graduates from any discipline with no previous clinical experience would not be appropriate candidates for home care. Working alone in the field requires a level of sophistication and knowledge rarely found in a new graduate. A safe approach to recruiting professional staff is to require, *at a minimum,* one year of acute care hospital experience, preferably in medicine and surgery. Educational qualifications can be associate's degree, diploma in nursing, or bachelor's degree. Obviously, any nurse with a graduate degree, previous public health experience, and/or certification in community health would be a "real find."

*Licensed practical nurses,* or *licensed vocational nurses* (LPNs/LVNs), can be utilized in either certified, licensed, or long-term home care programs to augment the skilled nursing care being provided to patients. As would be expected, the LPN must work under the supervision of an RN. The supervision does not have to be direct.

For instance, the RN develops the plan of care (POC) for a patient who requires twice daily straight catheterization. An LPN can perform the procedure as one of the twice daily visits or can perform twice daily catheterization for four consecutive days; the RN then sees the patient on the fifth day to assess and evaluate the patient's status.

Two years of acute care medicine and surgery experience should be required for LPNs who would like to work in community health.

## Physical Therapists (PT) and Speech Therapists (ST)

Physical and speech therapy are considered qualifying services; therapists must be able to develop and coordinate a POC. A minimum of two years of experience in a structured medical setting (private physician's office or nursing home), acute care hospital, or rehabilitation hospital would be appropriate for therapists who wish to join a community health organization. Unlike RNs, the PTs and STs do have a universal education process. A bachelor's degree is the minimum standard for entry into the profession.

## Occupational Therapist (OT)

Although not considered a qualifying service under M/C regulations, OTs must be able to develop a POC and fulfill it independently. Occupational therapists have the same educational and experience qualifications as the PTs and STs.

## Therapy Assistants

Physical therapy assistants (PTAs) and certified occupational therapy assistants (COTAs) function much as the LPNs/LVNs do. They must be supervised by a therapist in their respective disciplines and do not independently develop the POC. If PTAs and COTAs are utilized, they should have at least one year of experience in an acute care setting. To be eligible to sit for a certifying exam, the educational standard is an associate's degree in the particular discipline.

## Social Work

Medical social work is not considered a qualifying service and has limited applicability under M/C guidelines. However, the myriad of social and economic problems found in community health requires social workers who are well-rounded and knowledgeable in crisis intervention, counseling, and entitlements. Much like nursing, social work has a variety of educational credentials. Master's in social work (MSW) and bachelor's in social work (BSW) are the two primary degrees; there is also a certification (CSW) available after minimum educational requirements have been fulfilled. Irrespective of the degree, any social work professional interested in home care should have a minimum of two years of experience in a structured environment—hospital, outpatient clinic, or community mental health service.

## Nutritionists

Nutritionists instruct patients regarding regular and special diets. As many patients need to alter their diets based on illness or disease process, the nutritionist educates them regarding food selection and dietary compliance. A bachelor's degree with a major in food and nutrition, one year of professional experience in a health care setting, and experience in normal and therapeutic nutrition are requirements for a home care nutritionist.

## Audiologists

Planning and providing hearing rehabilitation for patients, performing formal hearing tests, assessing the appropriateness of hearing aid devices, and instructing patients and care givers in the appropriate use of hearing-enhancing equipment and devices are the tasks of an audiologist. Although the services of these professionals are not extensively used in most home care agencies, when utilized they can be an integral part of the treatment plan. Audiologists must have a bachelor's degree in audiology and a minimum of one year of experience in a health care setting.

# Administrative Staff

Within the agency, administrative staff is found at several levels. The functions of management staff depend on the size of the agency and its scope of service. Often state health departments mandate the titles and qualifications required for these positions. Agency senior management must be familiar with and comply with regulations for recruiting and retaining qualified managers. Several categories of management personnel will be discussed in this section.

## Administrative Nursing Supervisors

Providing the day-to-day supervision, evaluation, and coordination of the nursing staff is the function of administrative nursing supervisors (ANSs), clinical managers, or patient service managers (PSMs), as they are known in some agencies. These supervisors participate in the preparation of departmental policies and procedures, make recommendations regarding the need for additional nursing staff, and if education staff is not available, orient new staff to agency policies and procedures, and clinical responsibilities. Two years of experience in a certified home health agency (CHHA) as a direct care nurse is required for these baccalaureate-prepared nurses. Nursing supervisors may also be responsible for case managers, discharge planning (intake), quality management, and utilization review nurses.

### Assistant Director of Nursing

Agency senior management may decide to hire assistant directors of nursing (ADNs) for individual departments or programs. For example, the agency's quality management and/or utilization review activities might be directed by an individual in this position. The agency's discharge planning and/or education and recruitment activities are other areas that may be overseen by an ADN. Nurses interested in a position of this type should have a master's degree and a minimum of one year of home care supervisory experience.

### Director of Patient Services

This position, which is the equivalent of a director of nursing, is required by most state health departments and all accrediting organizations. It is a senior management role responsible for evaluating and supervising the nursing management staff, participating in the budget process, recommending the appropriate number of staff required to provide patient care, and overseeing the overall operations of the nursing staff.

In agencies without designated departmental managers, the director of patient services (DPS) is responsible for management of the social work and rehabilitation staff as well. In agencies with discrete social work and rehabilitation departments, the managers of those departments report to the DPS. Agencies may also have a separate DPS for its CHHA and another for other programs. While programmatic needs are different, the job requirements and qualifications are the same. The DPS requires a master's degree in nursing or a related field, plus a minimum of two years of supervisory experience in a CHHA or home health agency.

### Chief Clinical Officer

Found in some agency tables of organization (T.O.S.), is the title of chief clinical officer (CCO). The overall management of clinical operations within the agency falls to this executive manager. The DPSs, managers of social work and rehabilitation services, and in some agencies, the manager of quality improvement report to this individual. In addition to the coordination of all clinical activities, this master's-prepared nurse, or physical therapist, determines the requirements for supervision of clinical staff, develops position descriptions for all levels of clinical staff, and may function as the agency representative in the absence of the executive director/administrator. While the director(s) of patient services at most agencies perform some or all of these tasks, more agencies are looking toward the establishment of one position responsible for all clinical operations. In addition to a master's degree, four or more years of public health experience are required, two of which should be in a senior administrative capacity.

### Executive Director/Administrator

The executive director of the agency, also known as the administrator, is responsible for the overall management, leadership, and direction of the agency. Additional duties of this individual include program development and planning, development and monitoring of an annual budget, and development of agency policies. This position requires a master's degree in a health-related field, and a minimum of five years of senior managerial experience in a health care program. Many agencies prefer nurses as administrators, and while this is not mandatory, it has proven to be an asset, particularly in the area of clinical management. Many nurses are complementing their nursing degrees with a master's in business administration (MBA). Educational credentials in both clinical and nonclinical higher education assure that both aspects of agency business will be effectively addressed.

### Rehabilitation and Social Work Managers

These managers are responsible for the daily planning, coordination, and evaluation of the activities of the respective staff members.

Social work managers must have MSW/CSW credentials and at least two years of home care experience. Supervisory experience, although not a requirement, is preferred.

The rehabilitation service manager may be a PT, OT, or ST, and must have at least three years of clinical experience. Again, supervisory experience is preferred.

# RECRUITMENT

Recruitment of professional staff may be approached in several ways. No matter what approach is used, the person or department responsible for recruitment must be familiar with the categories and levels of staff required in the home health arena and how they differ from traditional noncommunity health requirements. Recruitment activities common to any agency include job or career fairs, use of staff as recruiters, print advertisement, and use of search firms.

## Job Fairs

Job or career fairs have proven to be excellent vehicles for recruitment. Sponsored by local newspapers or trade publications, these events draw hundreds of interested professionals. Agencies send representatives to the fairs with handouts, videos, visual displays, salary and scheduling information, education and experience requirements, and a variety of promotional *giveaways*. Professionals interested in home care are required to leave pertinent information for a return phone call or perhaps are asked to complete an employment application at the fair. Follow-up is then done by the agency.

## Agency Staff as Recruiters

Word of mouth remains a viable recruitment tool and works particularly well with support and paraprofessional staff. Organizations may offer a recruitment *bonus* for each new hire brought in by a current employee. Of course, the new hire must successfully complete pre-employment, orientation, and probation requirements and prove to be an acceptable employee before the bonus is paid. Agencies having contracts or educational arrangements with upper-division nursing schools, or physical, occupational, speech, or social work programs may find students who express an interest in working for the agency. Upon graduation *and* successful licensure, the new graduate's qualifications, skills, and experience must be evaluated. As noted earlier, many agencies require a minimum of one to two years of acute care or supervised experience, with some public health knowledge preferred. All levels of field staff are expected to demonstrate independence, self direction, and autonomy.

## Emerging Disciplines

Changing federal and state regulations affect the scope of recruitment an agency undertakes. For example, recent laws allowing PTAs and COTAs to practice under the supervision of a licensed PT have created a new category of home care staff. Recruitment efforts formerly geared toward licensed professionals must now be broadened to include new and emerging categories of home care workers.

## Search Firms

Professional search firms can reduce administrative recruitment activities by identifying, screening, and initially interviewing candidates for available positions. Once the initial screening is completed, interview dates and times are arranged, thus saving considerable time for the agency managers. These firms are paid by the agency or institution if the candidate is hired; most agencies have found this approach successful, especially for administrative vacancies.

## Recruitment for Hospital-Based and Related Agencies

Many hospital-based or hospital-related agencies (see Chapter 4 for definitions) use the staffing department of the institution to locate and screen applicants for home health positions. After preliminary screening by the staffing department, candidates are directed to the agency to arrange formal interviews with the appropriate department managers. This process saves the agency from performing preliminary screening. However, some agencies find it more expeditious to control their own recruitment and hiring and have designated recruitment personnel. There are hospital-based agencies that combine both methods, perhaps utilizing the hospital recruiters for clerical, support, or therapy services while managing their own nursing recruitment. Agencies servicing more than one hospital site may find interinstitutional "bulletin boards" useful to post available positions.

## Recruitment for Community-Based Agencies

Community-based agencies, as well as hospital-based agencies, depend heavily on advertisements. These ads may be regularly placed in local newspapers as part of the classified section, or as part of special monthly or weekly health care supplements. Professional journals and union publications usually contain ads for professional, paraprofessional, clerical, and other support staff at all levels. Paraprofessionals may also be recruited via regional or local ads. Participation and response at job fairs further enhances the recruitment efforts of community-based organizations.

# DETERMINING REQUIRED FULL-TIME EQUIVALENTS

In order to determine the required number of full-time equivalents (FTEs), an agency must first estimate its projected number of visits. Administrators then determine how many FTEs are required to make those visits, taking into consideration revenue-producing and nonvisit time.

### Calculation Example
The following example will provide a process for making this determination. Assume that

- a standard daily panel of patients for a direct care nurse is 6 visits per day. Panel is defined as the expected number of patients to be seen by a *salaried* employee on a daily basis.
- a nurse working 5 days per week mulitplied by 52 weeks works 260 days/year.

However, in most agencies, staff nurses receive 20 paid vacation days and 12 paid holidays as part of their benefits package. The average sick time utilization for this example will be 6 days per year. Mandatory education (cardiopulmonary resuscitation [CPR], infection control, etc.) may take up to 2 days, and other nonrevenue time, such as regulatory requirements, inservice sessions, patient-centered conferences and other required meetings may use another 3 days, for a total of 43 *paid nonrevenue* producing days per nurse.

Therefore, by subtracting 43 nonvisit days from a total of 260 anticipated work days, the average nurse actually works 217 days.

217 days × 6 patients per day = 1,302 visits per year per nurse.

If an agency is expected to make 42,000 nursing visits for the year, divide 42,000 by 1,302 = 32.25 required FTEs.

This formula may be used for all professional disciplines, based on annual budgeted visits and the panel expectation particular to the discipline. Required panels usually vary according to service. Chapter 18 will address productivity issues in more depth.

# WHAT OUTSIDE FACTORS INFLUENCE REQUIRED FTEs?

Outside factors often influence the number of FTEs an agency requires. Changing federal and state regulations may indicate a need for additional staff.

For example, in November, 1993, the New York State Department of Social Service required all HHAs to perform fiscal assessments on all Medicaid (M/A) clients requiring home health services for more than sixty days. The state mandated that each agency have an assessor and an evaluator. Since the tasks associated with this initiative could not be absorbed by existing personnel and were beyond a clerical position, a designated nurse *and* social worker were hired by some agencies.

## Automation

Federally mandated changes in how an agency processes claims or submits bills can also affect the number of FTEs required. As an example, the recent shift towards electronic claims submission (ECS) has necessitated the addition of management information systems (MIS) and clerical staff for many agencies.

## Managed Care

With a high degree of certainty, additional staff will be required to evaluate and process the myriad of insurance programs that have appeared and will continue to appear as a result of health care reform. In the era of managed care, early hospital discharges, and expanding outpatient therapy, additional nurses may be required to evaluate patients to ensure safe, effective discharge planning and appropriateness of alternative health care environments such as home care.

## Community Demographics

Changing demographics, shifting population density, or increasing crime rates require agencies to hire additional support staff, including security and escort personnel. The increase in patient volume in certain areas due to immigration trends and economic factors will compel the addition of staff at all levels.

# WHEN TO RECRUIT

In most instances, recruitment is an ongoing process. As patient population grows, technology for home care advances, financial considerations become more pressing, and staff is lost to normal attrition, agencies discover that there is an ever-present need to recruit staff. Recruitment should begin at the first indication of an impending vacancy. This includes any anticipated leaves of absence, promotions, resignations, or prolonged illnesses. Filling positions as early as possible lends itself to a more seamless transition as incumbent staff vacate positions.

When new programs, initiatives, or regulatory mandates are identified, recruitment must be a vital part. For example, the development of a maternal child health (MCH) program involves not only recruitment of MCH nurses, but of therapists, social workers, managers, clerical support, and perhaps paraprofessionals. Recruitment must be aggressive, not only for professional staff but for additional clerical and support staff needed to process and maintain the volumes of paperwork. The paper burden placed on the home care industry by federal, state, and local regulations is enormous, and professional staff produce the bulk of that paper. Therefore if there is an appreciable increase in professional staff, there is a corresponding need for clerical support.

## Unexpected Staff Needs

Home care agencies often find it necessary and beneficial to contract out for all levels of direct care givers and associated support personnel when there is an unexpected surge in visit volume. Large and small agencies may purchase all paraprofessional services from local businesses as well. Purchased services and all they entail will be discussed in Chapter 20, *Clinical Department Organization.*

# CONCLUSION

In order to recruit an adequate, effective, and committed staff, agency administrators must be mindful of the agency's scope of service, short- and long-term goals, and the number of people it will take to accomplish those goals. All facets of agency operation must be considered, not only in the clinical arena, but in the area of support services. Recruitment can and should occur on an ongoing basis, leaving no stone unturned in the search for qualified personnel. An agency should have an alternate plan and method to supplement staff for unexpected volume increases.

## *Suggested Readings*

Hargis, C. L. (1990). *Team building.* Baltimore, MD: Williams and Wilkins.

Vos, R. A. (1993). The challenge of filling vacancies. *The Journal of Nursing Administration, 23* (4), 39.

# CHAPTER

## 18

# Productivity Expectations for Clinical Staff

Susan Craig Schulmerich

Productivity for home health agency (HHA) field staff is not universally defined in the industry. There are simply too many variations from agency to agency. Factors impacting productivity will be discussed. This discussion is not exhaustive, but can be used as a point of reference for development of unique standards for individual agency operation and budgeting calculations.

# AGENCY VARIATIONS

As discussed in earlier chapters, there are appreciable, as well as subtle, differences in the composition, leadership, and governance of agencies. It should come as no surprise that productivity of staff will likewise be diverse. These variations may result because of

- distance to be traveled
- inclement weather
- union contracts
- professional experience of the staff
- whether the patient encounter is an initial visit, recertification (recert), or revisit (ongoing)
- productivity efficiencies (such as automation)
- complexity of patient diagnoses and needs

## Geography Served by the Agency

The distance staff must travel between visits is usually equated to surface miles, which is appropriate. However, in an inner city where the availability of mass transit may be lacking, the surface distance traveled between cases may be short but enormously time-consuming. Conversely, in an inner city where there are a number of visits within a city block or two, the time between visits, if scheduled appropriately, will be minimal.

In rural areas the time for travel may have a significant negative impact on the productivity levels of field staff. Protracted travel time obviously decreases revenue potential. Also, there is an associated expense of mileage reimbursement to staff.

### Weather Conditions

Inclement weather, whether snow, hurricanes, or tornadoes, plays havoc with expected visit volume and productivity, which translates to negative revenue generation against budgeted expectations. One chief financial officer coined Mother Nature's effects on budget projections as *"bad revenue days."* When bad revenue days are not accurately projected, the end-of-year impact can be startling. If normal daily revenue is $20,000 and there are fifteen unplanned (unbudgeted) bad revenue days, the gross negative impact can be as bad as $300,000 at the end of the year. The loss of $300,000 does not necessarily have a corresponding expense reduction since staff will, in all likelihood, use some form of benefit time to offset lost wages.

## Union Contracts

Collective bargaining agreements may address expected productivity levels of field staff. If this is the case, there must be two provisions in the agreement to protect management. First, if the industry develops techniques, systems, or automation advances that will enhance productivity, then the previously negotiated expectations must be revised upward with no appreciable salary increase. Second, if a staff member covered by the agreement consistently falls below expected productivity levels, there must be some form of recourse for the employer, either an *effective* disciplinary process or some monetary reconciliation. Obviously it would be best if the collective bargaining agreement were silent on the matter.

## Experience Level of the Field Staff

Productivity during orientation, as would be expected, is below that of incumbent staff. By the end of the orientation and probationary period the staff member should meet normal expectations. If the staff member is unable to meet expected productivity standards, then the clinical manager must make an educated guess as to whether the professional will, with minimal effort from both parties, be able to meet expectations in a finite period of time.

To assume that professional efficiency and abilities increase with years of experience is not unrealistic. Increased performance expectations can be acknowledged in an experience scale with associated increased productivity levels. The benefit of this type of arrangement is that the staff member does not have to show improved productivity if he or she chooses not to; however, pay increases, more than across-the-board adjustments, are predicated on productivity and not simply longevity.

## Visit Type

As would be expected, initial visits are longer in nature than revisits. An initial visit is a comprehensive assessment of all physical aspects of the patient and the social and emotional environment in which the patient resides. Documentation time associated with an initial visit is usually equal to or *longer* than the actual patient visit. A discussion of methods to reduce the amount of professional time spent performing activities other than taking care of patients follows in this chapter, and later in *Future Trends,* Chapter 24.

Any process or procedure that will reduce the paperwork activities associated with a visit not only improves staff morale but has the potential to improve productivity. Redundant patient information, that information that is recorded *on every visit,* is a target of opportunity for improvement. Figure 18–1 is a reproduction of a revisit note that illustrates how redundant information can be formatted to be more *user friendly.* Automation of the clinical note is the ultimate productivity enhancer, but until the home care software industry has *the* product, traditional paper efficiencies can and should be developed. Successful clinical automation requires that a good paper system

# MONTEFIORE HOME HEALTH AGENCY

## NURSING CLINICAL PROGRESS RECORD

| Staff | 00 | EMPLOYEE NUMBER |
|---|---|---|
| Staff FFS | 01 | |
| Indiv Cont | 02 | |

**1**

PATIENT NAME (LAST, FIRST, M.I.)

PATIENT I.D. #

**VISIT DATE**
_/_/_

NURSE

COORDINATOR

| VISIT CODE | TYPE CODE | D/C CODE | CHHA | Rx | PAYOR OVR. |
|---|---|---|---|---|---|
| | | | LTHHCP | | |

PRIMARY MEDICAL DIAGNOSIS

PERTINENT SECONDARY DIAGNOSES

SURGICAL PROCEDURES

**VISIT REASON: ASSESS: PHYS COND** __ S/S Comp __ Knowl of Care __ **TEACH:** Med Cond __ Diet __ Meds __ Rx __ Other __
**CARE:** Wd __ Decub __ Cath __ Ostomy __ Med Prep __ Other __ **EVAL:** Rx Compliance __ Response __ Functional __

## COGNITIVE / PERCEPTUAL

**NUTRITION / METABOLIC** __ Temp __
UPPER GI : NSA __ WT __ Bl. Gluc __
Noncompl: Diet __ Fluid __ Dysphagia __
Anorexia __ Nausea __ Vomiting __ GT Intact __
S/S Hyperglycemia __ S/S Hypoglycemia __
Receiving TPN/IV Fluids (spec) __

SKIN : NSA __ S/S Dehyd __ Rash __
Skin Lesions __ Incision __
Suture/Staples __ Drain __

WOUND ASSESS : __

**ELIMINATION**
GI : NSA __ Last BM __ Bowel Patt __
Invol __ Constip __ Diarrhea __
Abdomen: Distend __ Pain __ Bowel Snds __
Rectal Bld __ Ostomy Func __

GU : NSA __ Freq __ Urgency __ Incont __
Burning __ Dysuria __ Anuria __ Polyuria __
Hematuria __ Cloudy __ Concent __ Odor __
Foley Funct __ Ostomy Funct __

SEXUAL : NSA __
Vaginal / Penile : Dischg __ Bleeding __

## ACTIVITY / EXERCISE

**CARDIOVASCULAR** : NSA __ BP __
Pulse : Rad __ Apical __ A/R Def __
Weak __ Irreg __ Palpitations __
Chest Pain __ Nk Vein Disten __ Fatigue __
Edema : RLE __ LLE __ Sacral __ Other __
IV/Central Line Intact __

PERIPH CIRC : NSA __
Pulses : Weak __ Absent __ Site __
Extremities : Cold __ Dusky __ Other __

PULMONARY : NSA __ Respirations __
Lungs : Rt __ L __
Dysp @ Rest __ DOE __ Orhtopnea __
Cyanosis __ Cough __ Freq __
Sputum __
Trach Intact __ O2 __ Inhaler __

MUSCULOSKELETAL : NSA __
Joint : Pain __ Contracture __ Swelling __
ROM Deficit __ LE __ UE __
Fx __ Cast __ Pin __ Bedbound __
OOB ad lib __ OOB/Chair __ WC Bound __
Amb : Walker __ Cane __ Crutches __
Endurance Limited __ Feet __
OTHER : __

**MENTAL STATUS** : NSA __ A&O __
Letharg __ Poor Judge __ Poor Mem __

NEURO : NSA __ Vertigo __ HA __
Syncope __ Weakness __ Tremors __
Paresthesia __ Paralysis __ Apraxia __
Poor Balance __ Unsteady Gait __

SENSORY : NSA __ Aphasia __
Slur Speech __ Dysphasia __
Blur Vision __ Diplopia __ Agnosia __
Eye Disch __ Ear Disch __
PAIN : __

**SLEEP** NSA __ Insufficient __
Excessive __ Interrupted __
**COPING** NSA __ Ineffective __
Inad Support __ Drugs __ ETOH __
**SELF PERCEPTION** NSA __
Dependent __ Anxious __
Low Self Esteem __
**ROLE RELATIONSHIP** NSA __
Social Isolation __ Fam Nonsupp __
**HEALTH MANAGEMENT** NSA __
Knowledge Deficit __ Low Initiative __
**VALUE/BELIEF** NSA __
Effecting Healthcare __

ADDITIONAL ASSESSMENT/EVAL

222

**NURSING INTERVENTION**

WOUND : CLEAN / IRRIGATE :

COVER :

RX / CARE :

**TEACHING :  Pt = P     SO = S     HHA/PCW = A**

TOPIC: Health Mangt. _____ Diet _____ Meds _____
S/S Complic _____ Diab Reg. _____ Stress Mg _____
Safety _____ Other _____
Comprehension: Gd _____ Fair _____ Poor _____
Motivation: Gd _____ Fair _____ Poor _____
Continued Teaching Needed : _____
_____
_____
_____

**NURSING ASSESSMENT**

_____
_____
_____
_____
_____

**EVALUATION OF PROGRESS TOWARD GOALS ON THIS VISIT**

Achieved # _____ Moderate Progress # _____ Minimal Progress # _____ No Progress # _____ Revised # _____

Major Change this Visit :  Y _____ N _____ MD Contacted _____ Pt to See MD _____ HHA / PCW / HA / HSKPR  Present/Supv _____

**REVISIT PLAN / GOALS:**

Work Toward Goals # _____ Change HHA/PCW Hrs to _____ Change SN Visit Freq to _____

*SIGNATURE* _____  *DATE* _____

© MMC HHA 11/92                                    FILE = C:\FORMS\MARCIA\HC485VN1.FRM REV 6 11/13/92

**FIGURE  18.1**   (Reprinted with permission Montefiore Medical Center Home Health Agency.)

precedes automation. After implementation of an automated system, paper backup procedures must be available in the event of a computer disaster.

Recert visits are similar in nature to initial visits with a significant exception. The social, emotional, and physical environment of the patient is already known. In the recert process, the patient is physically evaluated for improvement, maintenance, or deterioration of the condition that required home care. Any coexisting problems or diagnoses that have been identified during the certification period are added to the recert. Usually a recert visit takes longer than a revisit, but is somewhat shorter than an initial. Again, the paperwork requirements are burdensome and account for most of the professional time.

## Productivity Efficiencies

Included in productivity efficiencies are

- automation of clinical documentation
- automation of scheduling
- discrete service areas and/or services
- reduction of the time staff spends in the office

### Automation of Clinical Documentation

The importance of automation of clinical documentation cannot be stressed enough, as the reader may have already guessed! In order for an agency to be viable in the coming era of managed care organizations (MCOs), health maintenance organizations (HMOs), and capitation, reducing the cost per visit is a critical component of survival. The most effective method of reducing the cost per visit is to increase the number of visits performed per day without increasing personnel costs. Clinical record automation is a fundamental component of the equation.

### Automation of Scheduling

Unfortunately home care software providers have not developed a product that sufficiently addresses this operational requirement. Maximization of existing personnel is an important element in the productivity equation. For a busy agency (the term "busy" is subjective), managing dozens of field staff assignments is very time consuming without the assistance of a *user friendly* automated scheduling system. The technology is available, it is just a matter of time before an entrepreneurial software company addresses the needs of the industry.

### Discrete Service Areas and Services

Geographic clustering—for example, by zip code—of patients and staff will enhance productivity. A discussion of geographic teams can be found in Chapter 21.

Assigning staff to specific patient service needs, especially when those needs are complex, is another means of promoting efficiency and productivity. Highly technical cases, such as those patients on life support equipment (ventilators, infusions, and so forth), require care from staff members who are familiar with these treatment modalities. Inexperienced staff, or those whose skills are not sharply honed, will be inefficient in visit time utilization, which translates to decreased productivity. An added benefit of service-discrete teams is that the staff will have the opportunity to expand its realm of practice into a subspecialty within the specialization of community health.

### Reducing the Time Staff Spends in the Office

Waiting for assignments, paperwork, case conferences, or escort/driver service is unacceptable in the new era of health care reimbursement. Inefficiency and ineffective use of expensive resources will simply render an agency impotent in reducing the cost per visit. An agency that has an exceptionally high cost per routine visit will not survive in a capitated arena. It is incumbent on agency management to assure the operation heeds the *four Rs.*

- the *right* staff member
- in the *right* patient assignment
- at the *right* time
- with the *right* resources

## Complexity of Patient Diagnoses

The complexity of patient needs and care are dependent upon a number of factors, including:

- diagnosis
- age
- socioeconomics
- available support systems

If an agency *specializes* in particular diagnoses, such as developmental disabilities, AIDS, Alzheimer's or hospice, or specializes in age-related care such as pediatrics, productivity expectations will probably be different than in a traditional agency.

# PRODUCTIVITY EXPECTATIONS

Productivity will address *salaried* employees, not per visit or fee for service staff. Definitions of types of employees can be found in Chapter 17. The various professional disciplines have differing expectations for the volume of patients to be seen in a *normal* workday. For instance, a medical social worker (MSW) visit is assumed to take longer than a skilled nursing visit. Physical and occupational therapy visits are similar in time consumption to a skilled nursing visit. Speech therapy time is equal to or greater than other rehabilitation disciplines. As a patient progresses toward attainment of goals, as set forth in the plan of care (POC), the amount of professional time per visit should decrease. Unfortunately there is no published data on the amount of time expended per visit. As stated earlier in this chapter, there is a recognized difference in the amount of time spent in an admission, recertification, and revisit.

## Cost vs. Revenue

In traditional health care delivery systems (acute care facilities), professional disciplines other than medicine are viewed as *cost centers*. In home health care, the professional care giver is an individual unit of *revenue* production. Each time a field staff member is somewhere other than the field, the agency has lost an opportunity to produce revenue.

## Positive and Negative Influences on Staff Productivity

Anything that has a positive or negative effect on the number of staff and/or types of field disciplines has a direct impact on revenue.

Positive influences, which have already been explored, include:

• automating clinical records
• clustering patients
• appropriate scheduling of staff to patients
• reducing time spent in the office

Another positive influence is timely discharge planning on the part of the hospital. When an agency receives a referral with less than forty-eight hours between the referral and the discharge of the patient, it can become a planning and scheduling nightmare. As length of stay (LOS) in hospitals becomes shorter and shorter, the need to involve home care *very* early in the discharge planning process becomes more critical. With adequate notice the entire process is smoother and less traumatic for the patient, hospital, and agency.

Negative influences include

• discipline-specific shortages such as the cyclical nursing shortage that occurred in the 1980s
• strikes by collective bargaining groups
• mandatory education, such as in-service for the Occupational Health and Safety Administration (OSHA) blood and respiratory-borne pathogen training
• conference time with the case manager, team conference, or administrative conferences, and so forth

Management is responsible for identifying negative influences and developing strategies to address them. Strong consideration should be given to utilizing the continuous quality improvement (CQI) process to reduce or eliminate negative productivity factors. Who better than the affected staff to find solutions to perplexing and costly problems?

# AVERAGE VISIT TIME

There is no published industry-wide *average time per visit*. As has been stated throughout this chapter, productivity and all that it encompasses is unique to an agency and the area of the country in which the agency is located. Physical patient contact time in a visit is no different, and depends on several factors. Some that have already been addressed are

- experience level of the staff
- type of visit
- complexity of care

    Additional factors to consider are

- amount and type of instruction needed
- who is to be taught—the patient, family, significant other, or a combination
- barriers present that affect the delivery of care, such as the physical or psychosocial environment
- language barriers

Time and motion studies or patient classification data do not exist for the industry. This frustrates administrators who are trying to develop patient care standards for their individual agencies. Very simply, there is no regional or national benchmark against which to measure an agency's performance. At this point, and until there are published and *accepted* outcome measures, the financial performance of an agency is the only objective measure of its *operational* efficiency and effectiveness. Quality improvement activities will identify patient care issues requiring attention, which will ultimately translate to efficiency and effectiveness.

# STAFF-TO-SUPERVISOR RATIOS

In developing staff-to-supervisor ratios, one should consider

- experience of the staff
- attrition and turnover
- complexity or level of technology employed in patient care delivery
- utilization of professional *extenders* such as physical therapy assistants (PTAs) or certified occupational therapy assistants (COTAs)

If any one or more of the above are present in the staff pool, then the number of supervisory personnel needed will increase.

## Experience and Attrition

If the agency has a large number of inexperienced staff or a high attrition and turnover percentage, the demand for supervision and support is appreciable. Agency administration should consider a high turnover rate as a signal of a very serious human relations problem and expend the necessary resources to resolve the issues.

## Complexity and Technology

Patients will continue to be discharged from hospitals sicker and quicker. This means home care will need to expand its capacity in the high-tech arena. Until high tech becomes the *norm*, clinical and educational supervision must be available for patient and staff safety.

## Professional Extenders

Utilization of PTAs, COTAs, and licensed practical/vocational nurses (LPNs/LVNs) will be necessitated by the increased volume of patients expected to be cared for in non-traditional settings. As the acuity of a patient diminishes, but as the patient is not safe for self care, utilization of PTAs, COTAs, or LPNs will bridge the gap until the patient is ready for discharge. The use of professional extenders with appropriate supervision is also an effective method in reducing the cost per visit.

# CONCLUSION

The home care industry is still in the formative stage of becoming a *business* in the true sense of the word. As a whole it does not have standards for productivity, patient acuity, or supervisor-to-staff ratios. In part this is a result of marked geographic and operational differences from one area of the country to another. It is due to the lack of data and information within the industry as well. In part it is also due to the fact that until recently, home care was not considered a significant factor in the health care industry. These elements influenced the allocation of business resources away from home care, which in turn negatively affected the development of needed operational data bases. Within the next few years, as integrated home care automation becomes more the norm than the exception, there will be volumes of information available to determine the effectiveness of an agency. Until that time, the financial *health* of the organization will be the primary indicator of efficiency and quality.

## *Suggested Readings*

Braunstein, M. L. (1994). Electronic patient records: a key to the managed care challenge? *Remington Report,* August/September, pp. 14–16.

Coriaty, B. (1994). The next generation in computer technology has arrived. *Remington Report,* June/July, pp. 24–29.

Reece, R. (1994). Community-based health measurement program: a new opportunity for the home health industry. *Remington Report,* April/May, pp. 19–23.

The Remington Review. (1994). Home care growth outpacing industry. *Remington Report,* April/May, p. 13.

The Remington Review. (1994). Home care industry. *Remington Report,* April/May, p. 15.

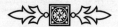

# CHAPTER

19

# Retention

**Stephanie Taylor Davis**

Although good recruitment efforts yield an adequate number of staff members, agency administration must also focus its efforts on the retention of that staff. The human and financial resources dedicated to continuous recruitment and orientation as a result of high turnover can stall the implementation of new programs and initiatives, place enormous demands on administrative staff, and negatively affect the morale of remaining staff. As more focus is placed on customer service, both external (patients, families, referral sources) and internal (agency personnel), a high retention rate should indicate a high level of job satisfaction, which in turn translates to customer satisfaction. The advantages of a clear and well-planned retention program are many, and include

- increased internal customer satisfaction
- strengthened commitment to job performance
- improved delivery of care

This section will investigate methods an agency may use to improve retention among staff.

# PROFESSIONAL ADVANCEMENT PROGRAMS

Many believe professional advancement programs are designed solely to move staff into managerial positions. Although that *is* one of the more common ways to reward and recognize superior performance and significant contribution to an organization, promotion is not necessarily everyone's goal. Professional advancement programs were first introduced in the acute care setting to retain a shrinking pool of clinicians. The programs that have been developed can be adapted to home care.

## Career Ladder Programs

Career, or clinical, ladder programs allow staff to retain current job functions while enjoying not only monetary gain, but greater autonomy in practice and a more diversified participation in agency activities. In a sample home care model, nursing staff may be divided into numerical or alphabetical categories, with differing productivity standards and qualifications for each. Nurses at a higher level might be required to publish professional articles or present in-service offerings on a particular topic. Nurses participating in this program would not be considered administrative personnel, but would be expected to orient new staff, participate in the development of orientation criteria, and assist in orientee evaluation.

A professional advancement program is also appropriate for rehabilitation and social work staff. Many organizations have therapists and/or social workers performing at different levels based on their willingness and ability to orient new staff, share information with peers, and, of course provide exemplary patient care.

One of the goals of a professional advancement program should be the development of standards of professional practice and the design of *caremaps,* or critical paths. A caremap is a multidisciplinary, measurable set of prescribed care activities and expected outcomes to be attained in a specified time frame. These may be based on diagnosis, length of stay (LOS), age, or any other identifiable factor. Utilizing "expert" advanced practice staff to develop the professional standards will add to the probability of acceptance and success when implemented. Administration must take several factors into account when developing and proposing clinical ladder programs. These include

- productivity expectations for each level. Will the highest category of staff visit more, less, or an equal number of patients as those staff members not participating in the program?
- salary differentials. Will staff participate for financial gain, professional growth, or both?
- additional responsibilities. Will there be requirements for publication, participation in regularly scheduled inservice presentations, or standards development?
- mandatory or voluntary nature of the program. Will this program be based solely on the staff member's desire to participate, or will staff be *required* to participate? Will the advancement program only affect new hires?

However career or clinical ladder programs are developed, guidelines must be clearly presented and a comprehensive overview of management and staff's responsibilities conducted. These programs, which are being implemented by a growing number of agencies, must be administered equitably and monitored frequently to assure the program is contemporary in the changing health care environment.

## Certification

Another method by which clinical advancement may be accomplished is through clinical certification. Many agencies recognize, either monetarily or otherwise, those staff members who are certified in a particular area of patient care or clinical practice. Certifying examinations are usually given annually; management should encourage staff to apply for these credentials. Enticements may include offering a paid day to sit for the examination, reimbursement for examination fees, or both.

Nursing has many specialty certifications that span all ages and practice areas. There is a community health nurse certification as well as medicine and surgery certification, which are appropriate for generic home care. Professional rehabilitation organizations offer specialized or certificate courses in specific treatment modalities. Social work professional organizations also offer certification examinations in particular aspects of mental health care such as pediatric, geriatric, or psychiatric care.

## MONETARY COMPENSATION

In today's environment of rising costs, albeit inflation has not been out of control, a competitive salary package can be one of the most important factors in the retention of staff. Agency administration must keep abreast of current salary trends and make every effort to remain competitive in the labor marketplace. In unionized organizations, salaries are determined through labor management negotiations at the time of contract renewal. In nonunion environments the salary package is determined by the financial and clinical management and the local job market.

# SHARED GOVERNANCE

Staff members who feel they are participating in the decision making process of the agency are more likely to remain loyal to that organization. Administrators should encourage staff participation in policy and standards development, and when feasible, should include a staff representative on standing agency committees. If appropriate, staff recommendations made during these meetings should be incorporated into minutes and then into practice. Staff input should be sought when decisions regarding program development are being made. Participation in the development of forms or the evaluation of new products and equipment are excellent opportunities to initiate staff into the decision making process. As is so often true, the best ideas come from the members of the organization who will be affected or use a product the most. The example in Chapter 7 of the dietary aide who saved the organization an appreciable expense and operational change illustrates this.

# PROGRESSIVE BENEFITS PACKAGE

While an attractive salary is a definite factor in the retention of staff, a comprehensive benefits package can be equally important. Family coverage, at a reasonable out-of-pocket cost, might be a pivotal factor from a single parent's point of view. A sampling of benefit categories an agency may wish to offer follows.

## Medical Benefits

Medical benefits include full or partial coverage for physician's office visits, hospitalizations, surgical procedures, maternity-related care, and diagnostic testing and screening for the employee and his or her dependents.

## Dental Benefits

Dental benefits include full or partial coverage for dental procedures and diagnostic evaluations. Coverage may vary to include orthodontia and cosmetic dentistry for the employee and family.

## Mental Health

Progressive benefits packages may provide full or partial coverage for psychological, psychiatric, or counseling services for employees and dependents. Many agencies have formal employee assistance programs (EAPs) where staff may receive individual counseling for assistance with work-related or personal matters. This service is provided free of charge to an employee and usually does *not* cover dependents unless the problems involve and have a direct relationship to an immediate family member. If an agency does not have a formal EAP, the department responsible for personnel management should refer employees to outside resources as needed.

## Automobile Allowance

Staff members who are required to use their own cars during the course of agency business are generally reimbursed for expenses incurred. The reimbursement rate is subject to current Internal Revenue Service (IRS) guidelines regarding mileage reimbursement, local automobile insurance costs, as well as by the amount of general wear and tear on the vehicle. The reimbursement is designed to offset those expenses and may be paid on a cost-per-mile basis or an average monthly allowance determined by category of employee, projected number of visits per day, or contractual obligations.

## Vacation/Holiday/Sick Time

Paid time off is another significant factor as a condition of employment. Agencies should be aware of, and competitive with, the local market for vacation days, holidays, and sick days granted per year. An emerging trend in benefit time is to group all paid time off into a pool of days the employee may use at his or her discretion. The days can be used for vacation, holiday, personal business, or family emergencies. In a predominantly female profession such as nursing, this has become a very attractive benefit. Discretionary use of time *on an unplanned basis* can cause havoc in the organization. If discretionary time is implemented, there must be very clear guidelines regarding what percentage of time can be used for unplanned absences.

Vacation time is usually a benefit that grows in direct proportion to the amount of time worked for an agency. In many agencies vacation time increases with the number of years an employee has worked. Also, seniority will most likely guarantee the choice of time off for vacations.

Paid time off may also include maternity, paternity, or adoption leave, marriage, and bereavement leave. The amount of time and under what circumstances an employee may use the benefit must be communicated to the staff at the time of orientation.

## The Changing Family Unit

In the current environment, the definition of a family unit has changed from the traditional nuclear unit to one that may include significant others, relatives, and life partners. Truly progressive packages, which are being offered by an increasing number of organizations, have extended medical and other benefits to companions and life partners. Administrators must consider alternate lifestyles when developing or implementing benefit packages and what the costs associated with these enriched benefits will be.

# RECOGNITION OF ACCOMPLISHMENTS

Staff members need to feel their accomplishments are known, appreciated, and shared. Such recognition can elevate morale, improve communication, encourage accomplishments of others who wish to be recognized, and enhance retention. Staff recognition can be accomplished in several ways, which include *written communication, oral communication,* and *creative communication.*

## Written Communication

Staff members who have completed a particularly difficult task, successfully managed a complex patient, or assisted with a difficult project may be recognized either by a formal individual note of thanks, a copy of which should go into the personnel file, or by a feature in the agency's newsletter or bulletin, if one exists. If the accomplishment is of particular interest to the affiliated hospital, parent company, or the industry as a whole, copies of the letter with a summary of the staff member's accomplishment should be sent to the appropriate persons for publication.

The annual performance appraisal should include acknowledgment of the employee's exemplary contribution to the agency and the profession. This documentation should address the positive impact the employee's actions had on the agency, whether financial, professional, or patient-related.

## Oral Communication

Accomplishments of personnel should be noted at department or team meetings. If the agency has general staff meetings, such achievements should be announced at that meeting and perhaps, if warranted, some type of award or memento presented. These awards may be for perfect attendance, assistance with a survey, or overall commitment to patient care. For example, the annual presentation of a director's or president's award for exceptional patient care or support service may be given and publicized throughout the organization. However employees are recognized, the formal and public notice goes a long way in keeping morale and motivation high.

Yet another way to recognize staff is through the practice of a formal, planned staff recognition day. Planned at the beginning of the year, this day may be celebrated with a breakfast or lunch, and by the distribution of small, useful items, such as fanny packs, umbrellas, or t-shirts with the company logo.

## Creative Communication

Agencies should consider new or unusual ways to communicate with staff. Production of an internal newsletter filled with information directly related to the events and personnel of the agency may not be unique but the layout certainly can be. Redesign should be considered at least once a year to keep interest in the publication peaked. In addition to the standard items about health care practice and cost containment, this newsletter may have "homey news"—announcements of births, marriages, condolences, get-well wishes, welcome messages to new staff, staff changes, promotions, and birthday greetings. A message from the executive director, agency president, or senior management representative should be an integral part of the publication. The newsletter must be published regularly *and on time.* The newsletter will lose its appeal if publishing deadlines are missed or ignored. Timeliness prevents news items from becoming stale and their impact diluted. A theme for each issue, which the feature articles bring together, and a "lighter side" section should be considered for basic format.

### Radio Station

If the agency has access to a public address system, this can be used to create an agency radio station. Current events and future plans relevant to agency operations can be presented as news bulletins. Additionally, a "radio station" allows timely dissemination of information and announcements that can then be followed up in the newsletter.

### Wall of Fame

Finally, in addition to announcing and writing about new employees, post pictures of new staff members in common areas where large numbers of staff congregate. Pictures of agency events and those staff who have notable accomplishments can be posted, too. In this instance, one picture is truly worth a thousand words.

## MORALE BUILDING PROGRAM

Agency administration must keep its fingers on the "morale pulse." If there are indications of a lowering of morale, then actions to rectify the actual or perceived issues must be taken. Honest, clear, *and timely* communication can be the solution to correcting misinformation and short-circuiting the agency rumor mill. Regularly scheduled meetings between agency staff and management will facilitate a sharing of ideas, renew commitment to the goals of the agency, and foster a willingness to solve identified problems.

### Customary Meetings

Monthly labor management meetings can bring concerns to the table before they become issues. Information gained at these meetings can then be relayed to the staff. Monthly meetings with various levels of staff help demonstrate that administration is involved and concerned not only with the agency as a whole, but with the needs of departments and individuals as well. Administration must be accessible to staff, either through an "open door" policy or by scheduling more formal appointments. Staff who feel administration is unapproachable or unconcerned will feel undervalued, overutilized, and unappreciated. Any number of resources, including Chapter 7 in this text, acknowledge the importance and impressive value of open, honest, and frequent communication between management and labor.

# SOCIAL EVENTS

Whenever possible, management personnel should participate in agency events, recognizing that social events are often the breeding ground for new ideas, suggestions, and improved relationships.

## Positive Reinforcement

In general, employees complain they are not praised enough when things go right, but never missed when things go wrong. *The One Minute Manager* by Kenneth Blanchard and Spencer Johns is an easy to read, commonsense guide to positive and negative reinforcement and is highly recommended for repeated reading. A little truly goes a long way when it comes to positive reinforcement. Managers would do well to keep this in mind, and remember to acknowledge staff as allowed, based on how formal or informal the climate of the agency and management style.

# CONTINUING EDUCATION

Full or partial reimbursement for continuing education offerings, tuition expenses for applicable advanced degree, and preparation courses for certifying examinations attracts many staff. Providing a particular degree is not a requirement for a position, salary increases may be given for formal education achievements. In a unionized environment, educational differential payment schedules are made during contract negotiations. Certification differential is administered much the same as education. Reasonable expenses associated with attendance at continuing education seminars, for example, food and travel costs, are reimbursable by most agencies.

# CONCLUSION

Low turnover rates among staff can only enhance an agency's ability to provide quality care. A stable staff is a confident one, and that confidence is projected to patients and peers alike. The consistency afforded the agency is invaluable, and administration will only profit from the resultant reduction of costs associated with overtime, recruitment activities, and lost revenue. Retention and morale must not be overlooked as an agency desires to "grow" programs and maintain a competitive edge.

# REFERENCES

Blanchard, K., Johns S. (1981). *The one minute manager.* New York Berkley Books.

# Suggested Readings

Bauer, M., Cherry, R. J., Clutter, P., Nelson, B., & Sandwell, A. (1993). Retention can be improved. *Nursing Management, 24* (10), 39–46.

de Savorgnani, A. A., Haring, R. C., & Galloway, S. (1993). Recruiting and retaining registered nurses in home healthcare. *Journal of Nursing Administration, 23* (6), 42–46.

National Institute of Business Management, Inc. (1993). *Creating and motivating a superior loyal staff,* New York, N.Y.: Brian W. Smith.

Schulmerich, S. C. (1993). An analysis of job morale factors of community health nurses who report a low turnover rate: A nurse executive responds. *Journal of Nursing Administration, 23* (6), 27–28.

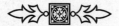

# CHAPTER

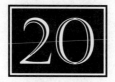

# Employment Process

**Stephanie Taylor Davis**

Before an agency can accept candidates for positions within the organization, determination must be made regarding whether those candidates are eligible for employment and competent to perform the tasks expected of them. Verification of applicable professional licenses, experience, driver's licenses and necessary automobile insurance, and relevant health information must be obtained and reviewed. Also, the areas of verbal, written, and interpersonal communication skills should be assessed. This chapter will discuss ways to determine eligibility for employment, and strategies to make the orientation process both meaningful and effective. The reader is directed to access any number of personnel management texts that address equal opportunity and guidelines for hiring the disabled.

# EMPLOYMENT PROCESS

When a candidate inquires about a particular position, information including specific job requirements, licensure, and experience should be offered. If an agency uses the recruitment department of an affiliated hospital or parent company, the licenses, professional registration, and educational credentials can be verified by that department. If the agency itself assumes this function, the task should be performed by a designated person with some background in human resources. The essential items required for employment in most home health agencies (HHAs) will be addressed in this section.

## Determination of Eligibility

Agencies look at many factors such as *licensure, health status, education and so forth,* when determining eligibility for employment. A discussion of several of these factors follows.

## Professional Licensing

All professionals, including nurses, therapists, and social workers, require valid licenses and current registration to practice. Prior to hiring, the person responsible for verifying credentials must see the actual license and/or registration; *copies should not be accepted.* If questions arise regarding the validity of any license or registration, the appropriate state licensing or education agency must be contacted. It is of the utmost importance that licensing agencies be immediately notified of any actual or suspected fraudulent use of a professional license. Candidates for employment must then correct any deficiencies or clarify any discrepancies prior to being hired. Incumbent staff face similar requirements regarding their credentials. Managers or the human resources department must implement procedures to systematically check that registrations have been renewed according to local law. Staff who do not renew in the prescribed time period cannot be permitted to work. The need for careful review of professional staff credentials applies equally to full-time, part-time, fee for service, and contract personnel.

### Paraprofessional Staff

Valid certificates from the appropriate training programs are required in order for a paraprofessional (home health aide or personal care assistant) to be eligible to care for patients. The agency must establish a consistent process for auditing the credentials of staff who work directly for a vendor agency. This can be done by on-site surveys of the vendor agency conducted by the agency's administrative or quality management staff, by review of documentation sent to the agency by the vendor, or both. In any case, paraprofessional credentials must be regularly examined to ensure the competency of those individuals.

## Health Requirements

Before patient contact, all staff must comply with state and federal guidelines regarding immunization and employee health status.

### Tuberculin Testing and Immunization

Tuberculin testing must be performed and documented at least annually, and more often for those professionals in high-risk categories, such as direct care nurses. Documented proof of immunity to measles and rubella must also be presented, either in the form of physician documentation, proof of immunization, and/or blood results.

### Employee Health Status

Staff members need to be in good physical health to perform their duties. Annual health assessments are required by accrediting standards and are useful in documenting new health problems of staff. Ideally these assessments contain questions regarding recent illnesses, medications taken, and treatment for any new illnesses. They should be reviewed by the agency's medical director or occupational health services department prior to incorporation into a secured section of the personnel file. Compliance with agency health requirements is a serious matter. If staff are noncompliant, actions must be taken, up to and including suspension from work with resulting loss of pay.

## Education/Certification

All formal education and certifications must be verified prior to hiring. Original diplomas, certifications, and mandatory continuing education attendance records must be presented and copies incorporated into the personnel file. All professional staff are required to attend an annual infection control update as mandated by the Occupational Health and Safety Administration (OSHA). In addition, clinical staff is required to update basic life support and cardiopulmonary resuscitation (CPR) skills every two years. Any items that are missing from the file or that have expired must be supplied by the applicant before a position is offered.

These standards apply to incumbent as well as incoming staff. The staff education department or human resources department is responsible for maintaining records of mandatory and formal education of the current staff, as well as the orientation records of newly hired personnel. An automated personnel system is invaluable in maintaining this information, particularly for agencies with large numbers of staff. These personnel systems are not, and probably should not be, part of the automated business/clinical system. If they are part of the business system, the files must be password protected. There are a number of commercially available stand-alone systems on the market.

## Experience

Most HHAs prefer that direct field staff have previous home care experience. This experience may be verified through reference checks or by contacting the personnel department at the previous place of employment. The scope of experience must be discussed with the previous employer in order to gain a clear and accurate picture of the potential employee's skills. Detailed prior employment information has become more difficult to obtain. Today it is customary for previous employers to verify dates of employment only.

For nonclinical staff, experience must be verified and references checked. While most clerical positions do not require previous home care experience, general, business office, and communication skills must be investigated. With today's increasingly sophisticated business and clinical automation technology, the competency of those who support the clinical staff must be of a level appropriate for the particular agency's needs.

An important facet of home care is the changing business environment. All staff—professional, paraprofessional, support, and administrative—must be adaptive and see change as a challenge and opportunity for growth.

## References

Two references should be requested for incoming staff. At least one of these references should relate directly to clinical performances or knowledge of basic clinical principles. References should address the areas of strengths and weaknesses, most recent accomplishments of the candidate, and the applicant's ability to work with administration, peers, and patients. Unfortunately, as stated earlier, many organizations will only verify employment dates. If this is the case, it must be made abundantly clear to the candidate that there is a probationary period during which time their self professed abilities and interpersonal skills will be evaluated.

During the interview process, the interviewer should get a feel for the candidate's knowledge, problem-solving skills, and understanding of the principles of home health care. Any questions or areas of concern should be discussed with the candidate and the opportunity for clarification offered prior to a positive or negative hiring decision.

## Additional Considerations

Candidates whose employment requires an automobile obviously must have a valid driver's license, car, and appropriate insurance as required by local regulations. Proof of these must be presented by the applicant. The agency should mandate proof of insurance as a requirement for auto allowance payments. A candidate without a valid license or sufficient insurance should be instructed to obtain the required items and return when this has been accomplished, *providing* all other requirements and interviews indicate this applicant is appropriate for the agency.

### *Americans with Disabilities*

Agencies must be cognizant of relevant laws pertaining to the hiring of employees with disabilities. Federal guidelines as set forth in the Americans With Disabilities Act (ADA) stipulate that employment may not be denied due to a person's handicap or disability *if* the handicap does not interfere with the requirements of the position. Agency administrators and those responsible for hiring must review this law carefully, and establish specific position descriptions that clearly address the degree of physical or mental acumen required for the job at hand. Position descriptions should include specific requirements—for example, the number of stairs staff may need to climb, the height of file cabinets clerical staff might be expected to use, and other specific, measurable activities relevant to the job. Of course, all civil rights codes must be adhered to when determining eligibility for hiring.

# ORIENTATION PROGRAMS

The goal of an orientation program should be to impart knowledge, and where necessary, alter or improve behavior. A comprehensive orientation program includes an introduction to the mission, goals, policies, procedures, job functions, and services of an organization. A successful orientation program will lead to increased retention and job satisfaction. This section will focus on the components that must be part of an orientation program and discuss what has been shown to facilitate learning.

## General Orientation

Clinical as well as nonclinical staff should participate in a basic orientation to the agency. This orientation should include a discussion of the history of the agency, the functions of the various departments and personnel, and a tour of the main office and the branch or satellite offices, if applicable. The generic overview should cover

- office procedures, such as work times and hours of operation
- sick and vacation time allowances
- resources available; for example, occupational health services (OHS), employee assistance programs (EAP), and education or training resources

- explanation of the fire, safety, and disaster plan
- policies regarding performance and health requirements
- policies and procedures for accident and incident reporting
- introduction to the management staff of the agency
- if appropriate, observation of field visits with all disciplines

## Professional Staff

Various literature on staff development identifies factors that facilitate learning and contribute to the success of an orientation program, thus leading to retention of staff. As identified in Chapter 7, the cost of orientation is impressive; therefore retaining the staff has a positive fiscal impact as well as a positive effect on morale. According to Leonard (1994), orientees report that the elements that lead to a successful orientation program are

- support by administration
- availability of educational resources and personnel
- an inviting feeling from incumbent staff
- small class size
- exemplary skills of the instructor
- a mixing of both formal and informal learning

Orientation programs must contain a process for ongoing evaluation to facilitate a smooth transition for staff who are more accustomed to the controlled hospital environment. Management must establish standards regarding how long field staff will stay on orientation and, in particular, how long the probation period is for inexperienced home care staff. Recommended orientation for experienced staff is six weeks. Those unfamiliar with home care should remain in supervised orientation for a minimum of eight weeks.

## Orientation Process

Within a prescribed period, new field staff will begin to make field visits, first with the educator or supervisor, and when appropriate, independently. Ongoing supervision and evaluation must be available if the educator or supervisor feels extended orientation is warranted because of identified deficiencies. An extension of orientation and/or probation must be based upon objective and measurable criteria. There should be a formal *performance improvement plan* developed, implemented, and routinely evaluated during the extension period. As unpleasant as it may be, there are times when the only alternative is to sever the relationship. When termination is required, sensitivity and understanding on the part of the manager can diffuse or prevent a distasteful situation.

### The Buddy System

To continue the orientation process, new field staff, or agency-based staff for that matter, should be "buddied" with peers after leaving the immediate observation of the supervisor or educator. This process, conducted through either a formal preceptor program or an informal buddy system, fosters collegiality and enhances team building.

## Specifics for Professional Orientation

During orientation the established professional standards for home health care, legal and regulatory requirements, an overview of the ethical issues that may arise, and the intake, referral, admission, discharge, and transfer processes must be clearly explained. The areas of risk management, quality management, infection control, and safety in the community require separate sessions with very detailed information.

For all professional staff, the role of the case manager, or home care coordinator, and how it interfaces with the direct care staff must be discussed to underscore the concept of coordination and continuity of care. Ample time should be allotted to the role of each discipline in relation to the overall plan, provision, and coordination of care, and discipline interactions.

A strong emphasis on confidentiality of information is important for all staff. With the advent of automated clinical information systems, patient confidentiality will become more critical. In the 1995 Joint Commission on Accreditation of Healthcare Organizations (JCAHO) manual, there is an entire section, and associated standards, for the management *and* security of patient information.

### *Documentation*

The area of documentation is probably one of the more important parts of orientation. The proverb "if it is not documented, it is not done" is particularly true in home care, where practice is so autonomous. Documentation requirements need to be taught, reinforced, and evaluated during orientation. The requirements for home care documentation are like no other segment of health care; clear explanations and procedures need to be a part of every session. Clinical notes should be evaluated by supervisory or educational staff and deficiencies identified immediately in the interest of developing good habits.

New nurses, and when appropriate, those in other disciplines, need a copy of the agency's medical relationship manual. Contained in this manual are policies detailing

- what services are available
- how and when to contact the physician
- what to do in an emergency
- medications that may or may not be given
- what actions to take in the event of conflicting or unusual orders
- care of the dying patient
- outlines of information to be included on initial visit documentation

This manual, along with a standard reference handbook of home health nursing or a discipline-specific reference text should be distributed to direct care staff at the time of orientation.

## Quality Improvement

The role of quality (management)improvement (QI) must be discussed with new staff so they will understand that *all* they do is considered QI and part of the continuous quality improvement (CQI) initiative of the agency. Staff members must feel free and *comfortable* to request QI evaluation of any topic they feel needs attention. Quality improvement staff should participate in every orientation to address not only documentation but the CQI program.

## Regulations and Payers

New staff must be cognizant of the rules and regulations of the various regulatory bodies. The requirements of Medicare, Medicaid, and private carriers for qualifying home care needs must be presented as part of the orientation. What constitutes and qualifies a patient for charity care should also be discussed.

## Fee for Service Orientation

Fee for service, or per diem, staff who have previous experience and are currently active do not require a basic practice orientation. Current is defined as actively employed in home care within the last six months. However, they do require an orientation to the unique policies, procedures, and documentation requirements of the agency. Attendance at an in-service program prior to receiving cases is mandatory. Included in this abbreviated orientation program are didactic sessions, field observation, and a supervised home visit.

## Physician Orientation

Some agencies have arrangements with intern or residency programs to provide education and observation visits to physicians in training. These doctors visit the agency for an overview of home care services and then accompany field staff on home visits. The objectives are to equip the physicians with an understanding of the needs of home care clients, the intricacies of home care regulations, and the importance of signing plans of care. Although not widely practiced, agencies that have participated in a physician training program report satisfaction on the part of the doctors, who express how much they have learned; the field staff who enjoy teaching what they know and do; and the patients, who are excited to have doctors in their homes.

# NONPROFESSIONAL STAFF ORIENTATION

As with other staff, those in new nonprofessional categories receive the general orientation and then participate in an orientation specific to their areas. Most orientation and training for this group is done by the appropriate manager and must include how the support function has a direct impact on patient care. When the new staff members' performance has been evaluated and is considered acceptable, they can assume their functions independently. The program content of job-specific orientation is distinctive and does not lend itself to "cookbook" development. Each agency will develop and modify these programs as necessary to meet operational needs.

# CONCLUSION

Effective orientation programs exist to facilitate learning and meet the goals and objectives of the organization. Administrators must be cognizant of factors that enhance learning. Orientation can then be the most effective tool in the quest for low turnover and true job satisfaction. Orientation never really ends; it is a continuous process through staff development. The positive impact of a comprehensive continuing education program is crucial in attaining a low attrition rate, which translates to quality patient care and organizational improvement.

## *Suggested Readings*

Cherry, C., Gartner, M., & Twardon, C. (1993). A competency achievement orientation program: Professional development of the home health nurse. *Journal of Nursing Administration, 23* (7/8) 20–25.

*Employee Relations Bulletin.* (1992). What the Americans with disabilities act requires your company to do. Report No. 1772. Waterford, CT.

Leonard, D. J. (1994). Factors perceived to facilitate and impede learning in the workplace. *Journal of Nursing Staff Development, 10* (2), 81–86.

Mangles, L. (1993). Model approach to hospital-based home health care orientation. *Journal of Home Health Care Practice, 5* (2), 9–13.

The Joint Commission. *1995 Accreditation Manual for Home Care.* (1994). Chicago: JCAHO.

# CHAPTER

# Clinical Department Organization

Stephanie Taylor Davis

The organization of clinical departments within an agency depends mainly on patient needs and visit patterns. Agencies may organize their clinical staff into geographic teams or develop diagnosis-specific patient care teams. However an agency decides to group its care givers, the primary goal must be the attainment of desired patient outcomes.

## EMPLOYEE STATUS

Before clinical organization can be addressed, the employment status of professional, paraprofessional, and clerical personnel must be considered. The types and definitions of staff can be found in Chapter 17, *Recruitment.* After deciding on the staff composition, full-time, part-time, fee for service, or contract, the table of organization (T.O.) for the clinical divisions can be created. The mix of full-time, part-time and FFS is dependent upon the operational needs, unionization, and philosophy of the organization. The federal conditions of participation (COPs) were changed in 1994 to require that the *primary qualifying* service of the agency be made up of employees of the organization. In other words, 100 percent of the staff providing the principal service delivered (usually skilled nursing) must be regular employees of the agency, as defined by the Internal Revenue Service (IRS). This new ruling will severely restrict the use of contractors for primary service delivery. However, FFS or contract staff can be utilized for the nonqualifying services such as occupational therapy (OT), medical social work (MSW), or home health aide (HHA).

Staffing a home health agency (HHA) is not dissimilar to staffing a hospital unit or any other patient care activity. The primary difference is that the patients in home care are not congregated in one area. The staff members in home care require the same consideration for vacation, holiday, education, and sick time as hospital staff. Here again, the difference in trying to accommodate for staff absence is more difficult because patients are not congregated in one place where there could be shared efficiency of staffing resources.

Within an agency staffing pattern, there should be full-time, part-time, FFS, and contract personnel lines for all disciplines and functions. The full-time staff are not particularly difficult to schedule, other than unanticipated sick time. The role of a part-time staff member is to augment the full-time staff. Fee for service is utilized when the visit volume exceeds the capabilities of the regular staff, or perhaps FFS is used to staff weekend and holiday visits. If FFS staff are not used on a regular basis, it is imperative the agency have some indication of when the FFS staff member is available for visits. It is not unreasonable to request a schedule of availability four weeks in advance of a particular date since the availability of these staff can have a direct impact on the agency's ability to admit cases.

## ORGANIZATION WITHIN EACH DISCIPLINE

The following example is a model often used to set up a patient care team. While it is by no means the only model, it has proven effective.

## Nursing Teams

Individual nursing teams are directed by an administrative nursing supervisor (ANS) who directs daily activities and performs general supervision of the team. Usually a team is divided by geographic areas, with the number of nurses assigned to the team being in direct proportion to the number of patients requiring service.

Depending upon the size and complexity of the agency, the ANS may supervise other disciplines or service-specific disciplines such as maternal-child, infusion, pediatric, and so forth. If this is the case, a very broad home care experience base is critical to the effectiveness of the ANS and the operation of the team that is supervised.

## Rehabilitation and Social Work Organization

In most instances, rehabilitation and social work departments are smaller than nursing departments, but that does not mean they cannot be separate and distinct from the nursing section. If there are discrete departments, they will usually be organized in a similar fashion as nursing, such as by geographic areas. Again, the composition of the department will be made up of full-time, part-time, and FFS personnel who will in all likelihood report to their own supervisors or managers.

# STRUCTURE OF PATIENT SERVICE GROUP

While each department functions as an individual unit within an agency, most have a common structure. This section will look at the team structure of several disciplines.

## Nursing Team Structure

Home care nursing teams can be comprised of an ANS, direct care nurses, and nursing coordinators. While most state health departments mandate some form of coordination of care, agencies are free to choose the team structure that works best for them.

### Admission Coordinator

The position of *admission coordinator,* or *admission nurse,* is utilized in some agencies. This nurse, responsible for admission visits

- assesses and evaluates the patient
- develops the plan of care (POC) for nursing and the personal care worker
- identifies the need for other disciplines
- begins discharge planning

These nurses report directly to the team ANS. If there are insufficient admission visits to fill a visit panel, then revisits should be added to the caseload for the day. Conversely, the number of admission nurses may not be sufficient to see all new patients admitted to the program. In that case, direct care staff will admit those cases. An admission visit consumes more time than a revisit, and visit panels should be adjusted accordingly.

## Direct Care Nurses

Revisits or continuing visits are performed by direct care nurses (DCNs). In agencies where admissions are not considered separate functions, DCNs are expected to admit, revisit, and discharge patients as needed. These nurses also report to the team ANS. For continuity of care it would be beneficial if the same nurse or group of nurses were to care for a patient. Aside from patient benefits, when primary nursing is utilized there is improved operational efficiencies and time utilization. Primary nursing is a model for the delivery of nursing care where one nurse is the principle professional care giver. The primary nurse is usually paired with another nurse who will care for the patient in the absence of the primary nurse.

## Nursing Coordinators

Most agencies utilize *nursing coordinators* to direct and orchestrate the various disciplines and services involved in a case. These baccalaureate nurses most often remain in the office, maintain regular telephone contact with patients, physicians, and care givers, and coordinate all facets of the patient's care. Information gathered by all direct care disciplines must be communicated to the nursing coordinator. The coordinator is the person who should have the most current patient information, and generally has the most frequent contact with the physician. Although not necessarily required, these nurses are encouraged to make home visits to assess the care given and assist with the implementation of the POC.

In some agencies, coordination is done by the direct nurse providing the care. However, the demands of effectively and efficiently coordinating the care of a group of more acutely ill patients, whose hospital length of stay has been appreciably shortened, has made it necessary for many agencies to separate this position from that of the DCN.

## Rehabilitation and Social Work Staff within the Team

Full-time therapists and medical social workers can be assigned geographically, as are nurses. Not only does it facilitate optimization of staffing resources, but it enhances teamwork among the members of the interdisciplinary group caring for the patient. Therapists and social workers, as well as nurses, are considered part of the team, although most patient service groups are described as nursing teams. Optimally, rehabilitation and social work staff should report to a discipline-specific manager. However, as noted earlier, they may report to an ANS in the absence of a designated discipline manager.

## Support Staff within the Team

Each team requires clerical support (secretaries and file clerks) in numbers sufficient to process the enormous amounts of documentation generated by the clinical staff.

These clerical workers report either to a designated business or support services manager, or to the ANS of the team. Clerical and support functions for the rehabilitation and social service departments may be performed by a secretary assigned only to the particular disciplines, or by secretaries within the nursing team.

When possible, escort or security personnel should be assigned and considered part of a team. Security service is usually geographic in nature. Therefore assignment of escorts by team would be appropriate.

### Paraprofessional Staff

In agencies where paraprofessional service is provided by employees of the agency, these personal care workers (aides) report to a designated nursing manager or to a support manager. These aides may be assigned according to availability, patient need, expertise, language compatibility, or geography.

Recently, as the result of cost containment measures by payers, *cluster care* has led to an increase in geographic case assignment. With growing frequency, aides are assigned to designated neighborhoods or urban area buildings in an effort to provide more efficient care and decrease travel and nonproductive time. Since there are state initiatives to provide personal care by clustering, agencies are well-advised to explore methods of assigning paraprofessional staff by discrete geographic area.

Some agencies, for reasons of unionization or training issues, have opted not to hire their own paraprofessional staff, but rather obtain aides from vendor agencies. These aides remain employees of the vendor agency, but are supervised by the direct care staff (nurses or physical therapists) providing skilled care. Aide service is requested by clinical staff and the referral facilitated by support staff (aide buyers) at the home care agency. When cases are accepted by vendors and aides, the information is conveyed to the clinical staff caring for the patient. Paraprofessional staff, whether employees of the agency or the vendor, are generally considered a part of the clinical care team whose involvement is commensurate with its responsibilities.

## Liaison Staff

The referral and intake of patients for care requires the skills of a nurse familiar with what constitutes an appropriate case for home care service. These nurses may be known as *liaison, home care,* or *intake coordinators* and work with the discharge planners, physicians, and nurses in the hospital or case managers from the payer source. They attend formal discharge planning rounds, and routinely visit clinics and outpatient and emergency departments to facilitate cases that are referred and ensure that the patient is referred to the appropriate provider. These nurses may report to a designated nursing manager or team ANS. While not considered a part of the nursing team, they must be part of clinical staff meetings and should be routinely represented at patient service meetings, case conferences, and quality management (QM) and utilization review (UR) meetings.

# INTEGRATION OF QUALITY MANAGEMENT/UTILIZATION REVIEW/RISK MANAGEMENT

Quality management, utilization review, and risk management (RM) activities are essential components of agency operations. These activities must be meticulously planned, coordinated, implemented, and documented. Accrediting organizations have increased their focus in these areas; agencies are advised to develop comprehensive programs encompassing *all* staff in the process.

## Quality Management

Quality management is any activity that improves processes, enhances patient care, increases customer satisfaction, or obtains desired outcomes. Agencies may have QM managers and staff, or assign QM activities to the staff of the agency. Because of the import and impact of QM/UR/RM, the likelihood of there not being at least one designated person for this function is remote. Whoever is responsible for the QM/UR/RM activities must either be a senior manager or report to a senior manager who is most often a nurse with degrees in advanced practice or theory.

All accrediting and licensing authorities acknowledge the necessity of staff support for QM activities; this support can be in the form of professional, clerical, or both, depending on agency size, complexity, and ownership. QM staff will participate in team meetings, patient-centered conferences, and the ethics committee.

## Utilization Review

Utilization review refers to those activities that determine if appropriate service was delivered in appropriate amounts. Cases not accepted for care and the reason for nonacceptance are usually reviewed on a regular basis at meetings required by local, state, or accrediting body regulations. Any staff or patient-related incidents or problems must be reported during the meetings. Utilization review meetings are conducted by either the manager of QM or another senior manager. Membership on the committee should consist of management and staff members; membership should be rotated to allow sharing of information and participation. Any deficiencies identified by the committee must be followed up on immediately with the management and clinical staff involved with the case. Issues of underutilization or overutilization of care should be addressed at the team level.

## Risk Management

Risk management activities may be shared by clinical management within the agency, but are most effective when coordinated by a designated department. In hospital-based agencies or chain organizations, this department, in conjunction with the parent company's RM unit, is responsible for the tracking, reporting, and follow-up of patient or staff incidents, and for providing appropriate RM education to staff.

Risk management personnel may be responsible for QM duties as well, and should be a part of any patient-centered conference where issues of safety, ethics, or practice are discussed. Likewise, RM personnel should be a part of the agency's ethics committee if one exists. Risk management activities should be reported at UR meetings and included in QM statistics and reporting.

## CONCLUSION

Whatever team structure is adopted by an agency, the goal should be the efficient and effective provision of patient care. Support personnel and support services must be included, when appropriate, in patient-centered conferences and integrated in the QM/UR/RM activities of the agency.

## *Suggested Readings*

Blau, J. M. (1986). *Administrative policies and procedures for home health care.* Rockville, MD: Aspen Publishers, Inc.

Lopresti, J., Whetstone, W.R. (1993). Total quality management: doing things right. *Nursing management, 24* (1) 34–36.

# CHAPTER

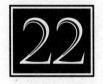

# Patient Admission, Discharge, Transfer, and Nonacceptance

Stephanie Taylor Davis

Federal conditions of participation (COPs), state regulations, and accrediting bodies require that agencies establish clear guidelines addressing what types of patients they can and will serve. Home care patients are an unusual population, and bring with them a wide variety of unique situations and concerns. This chapter will focus on some of those situations and discuss why clear admission, discharge, transfer (ADT), and nonacceptance policies are critical to agency operation.

# ADMISSION CRITERIA

Admission criteria must be consistent and easily understood by agency staff, discharge planning personnel, and all referral sources. In order to function effectively, intake staff, or those clinical personnel responsible for screening and accepting referrals, must be knowledgeable regarding the agency's admission criteria and act as resources to referral sources. Written policy and procedure, which should be reviewed and revised at least annually, outline the procedural process and criteria for acceptance. The policy should be distributed to staff during orientation and remain a part of the agency's clinical policy and procedure manual.

The policy needs to address

- when and how referrals are made
- what techniques are utilized by clinical staff in evaluating potential patients (interviews with patients, review of clinical documentation, home assessments)
- requirements for physician involvement in patient care

Also, incorporated into the policy are the catchment area the agency serves and within what time frames admission visits will be made. Significant consideration in determining whether or not to accept a patient for care will be discussed in this chapter.

## Patient Safety

For a patient to be accepted, the home must be safe and adequate for the delivery of care. Agencies may conduct preacceptance home evaluations to assess the patient's home environment. An assessment visit determines if what was seen during the in-patient setting resembles reality in the home. These assessments include

- an evaluation of telephone and electrical service
- whether there is running water and a clean place to provide care
- observations of the commitment of family members to caring for and having the patient at home

Patients should be self-directing and able to call for help in an emergency, and/or have an available, willing, and able care giver who can provide assistance and summon emergency personnel when needed. The majority of agencies require that an *accessible* significant other (S/O) be available and have ongoing involvement. With increasing frequency, agencies find themselves in the position of caring for an acutely ill patient with no family or friends nearby and no one to make decisions on the patient's behalf when and if the need arises.

## Initial Visits

Some state codes, as well as individual agency policies, stipulate that initial visits be made within twenty-four hours of acceptance. There may be exceptions to this rule—for instance, when the physician agrees to a later start of care, or when the patient or family requests a visit beyond the twenty-four hours. These exceptions must be clearly documented on intake records and scrupulously monitored.

## Scope of Services

Under the law, agencies can only accept cases they can safely and adequately service; the agency must be able to provide the services it advertises. Referral sources and patients have the right to expect and receive what is advertised. Confusion will be avoided if referral sources are aware of what services are provided by an agency *before* the referral is made. Intake documentation must include any special needs of the patient, as well as any other pertinent information that could affect the agency's ability to provide care, thus affecting the decision to admit the patient. For example, if an agency cannot provide a particular service such as infusion therapy or laboratory services and no contractual arrangement exists for the provision of that care, the agency is obligated to refer those cases to another agency with the appropriate scope of service.

## Nondiscrimination

Service may *not* be denied to patients based on religion, age, race, sex, creed, national origin, sexual orientation, ability to pay, location of residence, or service intensity. Also, service provided cannot be changed or reduced solely in response to changes in, or loss of, pay source.

## Patients with Complex Needs

An agency may implement policies requiring that patients with complex psychosocial and clinical needs be the subject of predischarge or preacceptance patient centered conferences. These conferences should include clinical and risk management personnel from both the in-patient setting and the home health agency (HHA). Any identified issues that could negatively affect the patient's home care course should be resolved prior to home care admission. If those issues cannot be resolved, the agency should assist in making alternate arrangements for the patient and remain available should the issue be resolved at a later date.

## Medicare Admission Qualification

Home care patients must be essentially homebound—that is, requiring the assistance of a device or person to leave home. Required services must be intermittent and restorative in nature. The development of reasonable and measurable goals geared toward improvement in functional status are required. These criteria should be regularly reviewed with in-patient discharge planners, intake and management staff, and other individuals involved in the referral and acceptance process.

# DISCHARGE CRITERIA

*Discharge planning from* home care should be started at the time of patient admission. The discharge *process* should begin at least two weeks in advance of the planned discharge date in order to coordinate the orders of the physician and the needs and desires of the patient. Obviously, documentation that reflects the coordination of all efforts is incorporated in the patient record. The establishment of realistic, measurable goals and the actions taken toward attainment of those goals can streamline and clarify the discharge planning process. Discussion of the criteria for safe and appropriate discharge follows.

## Patient and Staff Safety

As stipulated in state health codes and expanded upon in this chapter, an agency is not required to provide care where staff or patient safety is an issue. If agency personnel are faced with real or impending danger, or verbal or physical abuse, discharge from service is considered appropriate. Agencies must develop policies and implement procedures whereby staff members know when to contact their supervisors, when to continue care, and when to discharge the patient. Discharge under these circumstances must be discussed with all members of the health care team, including the physician, and a conference held to discuss alternate care arrangements. Options such as care in a safer location should be explored, and if necessary, the appropriate adult or child protective agencies notified. Patients discharged from service for reasons of safety should always be presented with choices regarding their care and ongoing needs.

## Noncompliance by Patient or Significant Other

Noncompliance with the treatment plan by either the patient or S/O must be accurately documented and discussed with the physician. Reasonable efforts must be made to encourage participation in the treatment plan and address identified barriers such as language, education, or psychosocial factors. Once it is determined the patient or S/O understands the treatment plan and continues to disregard clinical advice, instruction, and supervision, discharge may be indicated. With growing frequency, agencies utilize written contracts to formalize expectations on the part of patients or S/Os and the agency. These contracts, if implemented, indicate what behaviors will be tolerated by the agency and what behaviors qualify a patient for discharge. For instance, if the patient's family or S/O interferes with the POC, and that interference leads to a deterioration of the patient's physical condition or interferes with the attainment of therapeutic goals, the patient will have met the criteria for discharge.

An agency can develop its own forms with wording specific to the situation at hand, or use standardized contracts that may be available through the risk management department.

## Scope of Service

If clinical administration determines that the patient's needs cannot be met by the agency, the patient must be discharged or transferred to an agency or community organization that can safely and adequately meet the patient's needs. A patient whose needs have increased while functional status has decreased may need referral to a skilled nursing facility, or require a level of care available through local social service organizations. The agency is required to continue to care for the patient until such services can be implemented.

## Refusal of Service

Patients have the right to refuse service, request that service be discontinued, or ask that service be provided by another agency. Administrators and field staff should discuss such wishes with the patient, and if possible, correct and resolve issues identified by the patient. If the patient still insists on another agency, the physician must be informed of the patient's decision and the referral effected. The patient should then be discharged and all relevant patient care information provided to the accepting agency.

## Goal Attainment

Patients who have attained the therapeutic goals developed by themselves, the physician, and professional care givers have met the criteria for discharge. Goal setting must be realistic, measurable, and attainable within a specified period of time. Although most practitioners want to meet all the patient's needs, most often that is not possible, and care must focus on the most pressing needs in relation to the primary diagnosis. The fundamental goal of care is to facilitate the independence and safety of the patient, family, or S/O.

## Patients Not Found

It is strongly suggested that agencies develop clear policies regarding actions to be taken when patients are not found at home for scheduled visits. The policy should indicate how many times a care giver will return to a patient's home to attempt a visit and how the patient will be contacted to be informed of such visit efforts.

### *Notice to Patients*

The notice to patients should direct the patient to contact the agency for resumption or start of care. This notification can be sent by telegram or certified letter.

### Contact with Family or Significant Other

Family or S/Os, if known, should be contacted to determine if they know the patient's whereabouts. If the family or S/O believes the patient intended to participate in home care, then it would be appropriate to ask that the family or S/O enter the patient's premises with the care giver to determine if the patient is at home and incapacitated.

### Notification of the Physician

If the patient is not found after these actions, the agency must notify the physician that there will be no further attempts to visit. As always, timely, accurate documentation is critical.

### Action If an Initial Visit Has Not Been Made

If a patient has not yet received an initial visit, the discharge information (patient's address, phone number, next of kin, and expected discharge date) should be verified. Frequently patients not found at home for initial visits may not have been discharged from the referring facility. If the available information is correct and the patient has been discharged, a home visit should be attempted. If unsuccessful, the steps suggested above should be followed.

## Patient Is Institutionalized

Policies regarding how long patients will remain on program when there has been an interruption in service are strongly recommended. It may be determined that patients readmitted for planned procedures such as chemotherapy may be kept open for a pre-defined number of days. These cases only require updated physician orders regarding any change in treatment plan or medications, and acknowledgment of significant clinical changes that would affect the home care regimen.

Tracking mechanisms to locate the patient within the institution to assure the patient's return to the home care program should be developed. This tracking can be done either through the institution's admission list, telephone contact with the institution's discharge planning department, the agency's in-patient liaison staff, or the patient or S/O. If the patient remains in the institution longer than the number of days permitted in the policy, the patient is considered discharged. Established time frames for keeping patients *on hold* and how that information will be disseminated should be incorporated in the policy. It is entirely an internal agency decision as to the acceptable number of days a patient can be absent from program.

## Discharge Documentation

It cannot be stressed enough that whatever the discharge reason, clear documentation must be maintained in the clinical notes, the coordinator's daily documentation, or both to protect the agency and the care giver. Comprehensive discharge planning is the combined effort of the patient, S/O, physician, and, at times, the local social service or protective agencies. When all efforts to provide care to a patient have been exhausted and these efforts have been documented, an agency may discharge the patient without fear of violating regulations or the patient's rights.

# TRANSFER TO ALTERNATE CARE SOURCES

Patients who request or require service through another agency, or patients whose needs cannot be adequately met by an agency may be referred or transferred to another agency. Criteria for transfer and suggestions to facilitate that process will be discussed in this section.

## Transfer Information

Irrespective of the reason for transfer, there is patient information that will be communicated to the accepting agency. At a minimum this information is

- patient's current condition
- specific needs
- expected date of transfer
- a copy of the physician orders
- a summary of care and treatment(s)
- status of goals

## Patient Relocation

Patients who relocate and continue to require care at home need to be referred to an appropriate agency in the new area. Agencies belonging to professional groups, such as city, state, and national home care organizations, regularly receive listings of HHAs in various locations. These listings are complete with names of contact persons, addresses, phone numbers, and what services are provided. The referring agency may facilitate the transfer by contacting an agency to inquire if it is accepting new cases, or by asking the physician or patient if he or she has a preference.

## Patient Request for Another Agency

Patients may request service from another agency based on a previous history with that agency, an interest in a particular program offered by that agency, or by dissatisfaction with the current agency. The latter must be addressed by agency management immediately. If the problem cannot be resolved, the agency should then refer the patient to the agency of his or her choice. Patient transfer information identified earlier, as well as any psychosocial factors leading to the transfer, should be provided to the accepting agency and the physician.

Patients may also request or require a different level of care based on diagnosis or care needs. Home care patients are regularly referred to hospice programs, skilled nursing facilities (SNFs), or programs designed to provide specialized services to a particular population, such as pediatric or geriatric health related facilities or day care programs.

Patient wishes are always the primary concern when determining both care needs and who will provide that care. Agency administration should make every effort to facilitate a smooth transition from one care source to another.

# REASONS FOR NONACCEPTANCE

Although agencies must make every effort to accept patients referred, in certain instances patients may be inappropriate and therefore ineligible for home care services.

## Safety of Staff or Patient

Agencies are not obligated to treat patients who present a danger, either real or implied, to clinical staff or to themselves. Patients whose environments will not facilitate an improvement in status will remain ineligible for home care services. The term *unsafe* can encompass environmentally unsafe homes—for example, those dwellings that are dirty or cluttered, or without water or heat. It is also interpreted to mean those patients with inadequate social supports such as an S/O or available care giver to provide care when the agency is unavailable, or at the point the patient no longer has qualifying needs. Further, *unsafe patients* encompasses those whose needs exceed what the agency can provide. Discussion with the referral source and patient to identify an alternative home care or continuing care agency is appropriate.

## Patients without Skilled Needs

Patients who have primarily custodial needs do not qualify for service by a certified home health agency (CHHA). This category of patient would include those whose primary need is paraprofessional, or where no reasonable expectation regarding progress exists. A patient in this category requires maintenance rather than skilled, intermittent care, and should be referred to local social service departments or assisted living programs (ALPs). Assisted living programs often take the form of congregate housing, and may provide personal care services and custodial support.

## Patients Who Are Not Homebound

Patients who are not homebound and can receive care in a physician's office or clinic should be advised to do so, since they will not meet one of the qualifying criteria under the Medicare benefit. Of course, if the patient, family, or S/O wishes to pay the published charge, then consideration can be given to admitting the patient for a *finite* period. Such a situation should be carefully evaluated and considered on a case-by-case basis. An agency could find itself in a particularly difficult situation regarding abandonment if a patient refuses to pay after indicating he or she would. Examples of patients who are not considered homebound might be younger patients who attend school, patients with upper extremity injuries, or those who have reached their maximum levels of function and are safe in the community.

### Insufficient Agency Personnel

An agency may be unable to accept a patient due to inadequate staffing. If personnel resources are not available to provide care in a timely manner, the patient should be referred elsewhere. Delays in initial visits can lead to retardation of patient progress, and would almost always violate admission guidelines. Agencies may have arrangements with identified "sister" agencies to whom they can refer when they are unable to accept patients.

## RECORD KEEPING

Detailed record keeping regarding cases not accepted for care is necessary. The record should include the patient's name, reason for nonacceptance, and any alternate care arrangements made for the patient. With a high degree of certainty this information will be requested by licensing or accrediting organizations.

### Benefits of Nonacceptance

The reasons for nonacceptance can be utilized to defend personnel requests. For instance

- statistics can be powerful indicators of the need for more professional staff when the number of cases not accepted because of inadequate staff is translated into lost revenue
- cases not accepted due to reasons of safety or inadequate social supports may indicate the need for additional escort/drivers or medical social workers
- inappropriate referrals indicate the need for referral source education in admission guidelines

Statistics regarding cases not accepted should be reviewed and discussed at least quarterly. If the review identifies any commonalities from period to period, this information should be forwarded to the QI department for investigation and evaluation.

## CONCLUSION

An agency, through its administrators, is responsible to ensure that the patients accepted for care are appropriate for home care services, require the skills of professional clinical personnel, and will be able to make reasonable progress toward goals. When those patients exhibit signs of noncompliance, demonstrate unsafe behaviors, or require care in unsafe environments, the agency has the right and obligation to protect both its staff and the patient. In spite of the best intentions and the desire to provide care, patients have the right to self-determination, and the right to refuse care or request care from another source. Those wishes must be honored. Clear and consistently applied ADT and nonacceptance guidelines will facilitate an often difficult process.

## Suggested Readings

State of New York. (1994). *Official Compilation of Codes, Rules and Regulations.* Albany, N.Y.: Department of State.

# CHAPTER

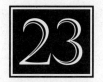

# Staff Safety Concerns

### Stephanie Taylor Davis

Safety of the staff working in the community must be a primary concern for agency administration. Safety issues are usually associated with violence; however, in community health, environmental dangers, weather emergencies, and vehicular accidents must also be considered. The focus of this chapter will be directed toward physical safety in an increasingly violent society and methods agencies may utilize to ensure and enhance that safety.

Unlike the more controlled in-patient environment, the home care arena is unpredictable, ever-changing, and subject to more external factors than most areas of health care. The security of personnel is one of the more frequently voiced concerns during discussions of home health; and it is, as crime statistics show, a valid one. Every agency must make a concerted effort to formalize its safety policies and to communicate those policies clearly and frequently.

# IDENTIFYING AREAS

Geographic areas requiring close safety monitoring are usually first identified by the field staff working in those areas. If the neighborhood in question has not required escort service before, security should be provided based on the staff's judgment, observations, and feelings regarding the situation. Additionally, local police precincts and published crime statistics should offer agency administration information regarding which sections of the community require security consideration. Local law enforcement units or community service associations should be contacted prior to agency start-up or before expansion into new areas.

Once areas are identified, the information must be quickly disseminated to staff, administration, and the department of the agency responsible for providing escort personnel. An agency may adopt a time-oriented approach to the provision of escorts; for example, escorts may only be provided after dusk or at a pre-determined hour. When areas are identified, staff must feel comfortable in requesting security service, and know their concerns will be addressed in the overall safety plan of the agency.

# COMPLIANCE WITH LOCAL AND FEDERAL ADMISSION REQUIREMENTS

In most areas of the country, state and local codes expressly prohibit agency denial of services to a patient based solely on the location of his or her residence (known as redlining). Federal codes also forbid discrimination of this kind. However, those same codes provide for the safety of staff facing actual or potentially dangerous situations. State codes, as exemplified by New York State Rules and Regulations (NYCRR:10 Section 763.5), do not require treating a patient ". . . when conditions in or around the home . . . imminently threaten the safety of staff. . . ." How then do agencies find the safest, most appropriate way to care for patients?

# WHEN SAFETY IS QUESTIONABLE

Staff members are instructed to identify those situations requiring investigation, notify their supervisors, and where possible, make recommendations to their patients for treatment in an environment that is more secure. If conditions in or around the home are contributing to the patient's unwillingness or inability to comply with the treatment plan, and therefore are hindering recovery, staff has a duty to refer the patient to local protective agencies. Of course, the patient's significant other (S/O) and physician must be notified and their input considered.

Multidisciplinary case conferences involving all members of the health care team should be held as soon as safety issues are identified. A risk management or quality management representative should be present to address any issues of liability relevant to the case. If possible, the patient and the family should be allowed to participate in the meeting. In-hospital bedside conferences should be held prior to discharge when it becomes apparent that safety for either the patient or agency personnel might become an issue.

## No Visit Address

Discharge planning personnel must be advised to scrupulously record accurate *and* current patient demographic information for the intake and field staff. An agency may adopt a policy of "no visit" addresses (not to be confused with red-lining), where care may not be given due to documented safety concerns. Such addresses may be abandoned buildings, no building/dwelling, or other places where care cannot and should not be rendered. Therefore accuracy of referral information is critical for acceptance of patients. Also, an agency may develop and implement policies regarding *caution* addresses, where visits can be made, but extra vigilance is required due to previous reports of unsafe conditions. Whatever the policy of the individual agency, arrangements must be made in conjunction with other members of the health care team to ensure that patients receive needed care in the safest environment possible.

# STAFF SAFETY EDUCATION

During orientation, staff should be given the policy and procedure regarding safety in the community. This policy, which all agencies must consider developing, must be reviewed annually and updated or revised as situations warrant. The policy should include procedures that detail what to do for unexpected behaviors and what are acceptable responses by the staff when confronted with an unsafe situation, either in the patient's home or in the community.

## Questionable Residences

Staff is advised not to enter a residence if there is any suspicious activity in or around the building. They should be advised to consult their supervisors, and if feasible, return later in the day. In large urban areas, issues such as nonworking elevators, enclosed and often darkened stairwells, and locked, gated foyers are all factors to be considered during the course of making a visit. Stairwells, where people may congregate for illegal activities, should be avoided. However, all reasonable caution must be taken when using elevators—for instance, remaining close to the floor/alarm panel, knowing the destination once the elevator is exited, and above all, trusting one's instincts regarding persons or situations.

Staff must be encouraged to memorize the location of public (working) telephones, police and fire call boxes, gas stations, stores, and other landmarks. The agency must clearly address the limits to which a care giver will go to provide care—for example, the number of flights of stairs staff can be expected to walk up and down if elevators are not working.

Staff members need to feel comfortable requesting an escort, even if escorts were not previously required. Sometimes a decision must be made not to enter a building at all. When making home visits, it is truly better to be safe than sorry.

## Personal Effects

Guidelines regarding what to carry on one's person, particularly in professional bags, should be clarified during staff orientation. *Fanny packs* instead of purses are a safe choice, as is the carrying of minimal identification, no credit cards, and only enough money to meet the day's needs. Male staff should be encouraged not to carry money, keys, or other valuables in expected places on the body; pickpockets have been known to anticipate, target, and victimize home care workers. Staff may need to bribe the gate-keepers or "unofficial security guards" of a particular building or neighborhood; this has sometimes been the only way to get in to see a patient and then to get out again.

## Vehicles and Uniforms

There are differing schools of thought regarding the use of identifiable agency vehicles versus unmarked cars, the use of street clothes versus uniforms, and the staff's need to blend into communities.

Many agencies encourage or even mandate staff to use their own vehicles, and do not require staff to wear a uniform of any kind. However, it is worth noting that in certain parts of the community, unmarked agency cars may be mistaken for police vehicles. More than one visiting nurse, therapist, or social worker has been wrongfully suspected of having business other than the provision of health care. Explanations regarding the true purpose of the home visit are sometimes required by the local gang controlling the area to ensure staff safety.

Staff members should be encouraged to keep their vehicles in good working order, be ever mindful of gasoline and oil levels, and have basic emergency equipment. Items such as flares, flashlights, fire extinguishers, maps, shovels, and de-icers should be carried and easily accessible. Although most visits are made during daytime hours, staff are advised to park cars in well-lit, populated areas. A convenient parking space is no substitute for safety.

In rural, sometimes isolated areas, staff must note access roads (primary and secondary), the location of and distance between houses, local landmarks, and gas stations. While car phones are not yet standard operating equipment, many agencies are considering these devices as safety and care enhancements. The latter aspect, care enhancement, is due to the fact that not all patients will allow staff to use their telephones, nor may they be in working order.

## Continuing Education

The agency should provide field and office staff with regularly scheduled safety programs. These programs may be given by local police officers, community safety groups, self-defense groups, or formal safety educators. Often these sessions provide hands-on experience, and staff is encouraged to role play actual or potential situations. Although field staff faces the more present and frequent danger, all employees must travel to and from work and live safely in their communities. Safety education should be provided to everyone.

# ESCORT/DRIVERS

Crime statistics and news reports regarding certain areas of the community identify the dangers faced by field staff member during the course of their visits. Because an area has not required escort service does not necessarily mean it is safe. Any part of the community can be hazardous.

Escort personnel must be utilized in any situation where the care giver feels apprehensive, unsure, or vulnerable. Escort personnel may be procured from several sources. Two sources and the advantages and disadvantages of each will be discussed.

## Security Services

An agency may execute a contract with an independent escort or security service. Often these organizations are staffed by retired (unarmed) law enforcement personnel. They escort staff into identified areas, using the staff's vehicles, and may accompany staff into apartments or homes while care is being given. If the presence of nonagency staff poses a problem for patients, the escort might be requested to wait in the lobby or foyer of the residence. Contracting for escort service provides flexibility by adding or eliminating personnel as the need arises. Generally the agency is assured a cadre of streetwise, knowledgeable escorts. Contracted escorts are not employees of a home health agency, but their activities require an agency-designated manager who will oversee contract negotiations, problem solving, and financial arrangements. Unfortunately the nonemployee status of these escorts does not lend itself to "teamwork," particularly if this type of service is used as a fill-in or backup service. The field staff who require escorts need to build a partner mentality with the escort. Not dissimilar to any two-person team, each will come to know what the other is thinking, and how she or he will react in a given situation.

## Escort/Drivers as Agency Personnel

Agencies may choose to hire escorts, either on a part-time, full-time, or contingency (as needed) basis. It is not necessarily a requirement that these escorts have formal security training, but it is expected that they be streetwise and comfortable in the community the agency serves. These escorts accompany the care giver into the patient's home and wait in a designated area until care is completed.

In all situations, the role of the escort must be explained to the patient, and the patient's wishes for security and privacy honored. These escorts are employees of the agency, and as such, are subject to the benefits and requirements associated with that employment. One advantage, often cited by both field staff and escorts, is that of comraderie and team building. Escorts and care givers may be scheduled together on a regular basis; some agencies may even pair the two in an agency-owned vehicle to enhance consistency for the driver and care giver. Often patients find it reassuring to see the same staff members on each visit.

All categories of escorts must have *clean* driving records, valid licenses, and no criminal record. The agency's personnel or human resources department should regularly validate and update this information.

## ALTERNATE DELIVERY SITES

Much of what has been discussed in this chapter involves external factors and focuses on events that may occur outside a patient's home. However, situations arise when the safety of the staff and patient is compromised within the patient's dwelling. Staff is not required to continue service when danger is imminent. However, there remains a duty to care for the patient. In these circumstances, and in accord with the physician's treatment plan, options must be explored. Patients may receive care at the home of a friend, relative, or significant other, and then return to his or her own home, if desired. If the patient has requested or is requesting a change of residence because of safety or environmental issues, the agency should provide appropriate services (e.g., social work) to facilitate this process.

Patients who are adamant about remaining in their own homes, even though they may be perceived by agency staff as being unsafe or inappropriate, may be referred for more frequent clinic or outpatient visits if a safer environment cannot be arranged. Although not recommended, patients have reportedly been treated in local taverns, restaurants, parks, schools, and places of employment or worship with no untoward effects; the question of homebound status must then be addressed. While every effort must be made to provide care to truly homebound patients, the care giver's primary concern must always be personal safety as well as the safety of other agency staff and the patient. Any unsafe or suspected illegal situations noted in the patient's home must be reported to agency administration and the patient's physician for appropriate follow-up.

## CONCLUSION

Staff safety cannot be overlooked in an environment that changes rapidly and unexpectedly. Agency administrators must encourage their personnel and risk management departments to provide both the education and the staff needed to preserve the safety of staff and the clients they serve.

## REFERENCES

State of New York (1994). *Official compilation of codes, rules and regulations.* Albany, NY: Department of State.

## *Suggested Readings*

Cohen, A. (1993). *Become streetwise! A woman's guide to personal safety.* Massapequa Park, NY: Target Consultants International Ltd.

Walcott-McQuigg, J. A. & Ervin, N. E. (1992). Stressors in the workplace: community health nurses. *Public Health Nursing, 9* (1) 65–71.

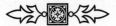

# PART FOUR

## FUTURE TRENDS

# CHAPTER

# Future Trends

### Susan Craig Schulmerich

The technology and financing of health care is changing so rapidly that what might have been thought to be futuristic a week or a month ago has come and gone. At a presentation by the Healthcare Association of New York State (March 1, 1995), Mary Jane Wurth stated, "The future is ahead of schedule." That statement succinctly describes the situation faced by health care administrators throughout the nation and the problems they face for short- and long-term strategic planning. The long term planning process becomes a roll of the dice as changes come so swiftly. Alden Solovy (1995) stated in an article titled *Predicting the Unpredictable*, "Throw out your strategic plan. Burn your planning handbooks. Health care is changing too fast for the traditional processes to be effective. Critical opportunities come and go in the time it takes conventional planning to gear up and identify opportunities."

In home care, with a high degree of certainty, there are four things that will happen; the form they will finally take remains to be seen.

1. There will be some type of health care reform, certainly on the state level and in all likelihood on the national level in 1997.
2. Home care will be a primary player in the *new order* of health care.
3. There will be an abundance of qualified professional, paraprofessional, and support staff displaced from the traditional hospital work force.
4. Automation within the entire spectrum of health care delivery will flourish.

This last chapter will explore the future, albeit with myopic vision.

# HEALTH CARE REFORM

Over a span of ten to twelve months literally hundreds of pages of material were gathered on health care reform in preparation for this text. In the later part of 1993 and the first nine months of 1994 there was an plethora of information on health care reform, which included

- who was sponsoring the legislation *d'jour*
- what small health care organizations were being acquired by large corporations
- what alliances and networks were being formed between organizations that heretofore had been competitors
- what new language of networks, partnerships, preferred providers, and acronyms abounded

Health care reform, and all the activities associated with it, were traveling at warp speed and headed for a brick wall. Health care reform and the brick wall collided in the fall of 1994 when the House of Representatives (where Representatives were all up for reelection), the Senate (where approximately one third of the Senators were up for reelection), and President Clinton (who was halfway through his Presidency) acknowledged that health care reform could not be accomplished by the 103rd Congress *before* the November 1994 election. The House, Senate, and President all pledged to make health care reform a reality in the 104th Congress.

## "WHAT A DIFFERENCE A DAY MAKES"

Election day 1994 (November 8) brought the Clinton administration's proposed *Health Security Act* to its knees and it would appear, to an end. Political analysts will debate for decades what the precipitating factors were that caused the American electorate to send incumbents, in particular Democratic incumbents, to the political unemployment line. As state and national political leadership changed, health care reform moved off the American public agenda. The changed agenda was in part a result of incredible market forces causing the health care industry to adjust itself in order to survive in a new age of consumer and payer demands and expectations.

### How Will Medicare Look in the Future?

By all accounts, the traditional fee-for-service, cost-based environment is on the queue for elimination. In an interview with *Health Systems Review* (1995), Ways and Means Subcommittee Chairman Bill Thomas (R-CA) said, ". . . This will force providers to compete for Medicare business based upon price and quality. Medicare recipients are consumers, and they're going to get more for their buck that way." For home health agencies (HHAs) this is a dramatic departure from the way they have done business since the advent of Medicare (M/C). Those agencies that can be flexible and cost-efficient and can quickly accommodate change will be the winners in the new era.

## THE INDUSTRY'S PREPARATION FOR HEALTH CARE REFORM

During 1993 and 1994, the health care industry began to take evasive action to ward off a wholesale disaster in the event health care reform, as had been proposed by President Clinton, became a reality. These actions included forming networks, preferred provider organizations, and alliances, or acquiring existing businesses, ostensibly to gain operational efficiencies. There was always the question of whether these actions were designed to reduce or eliminate the number of independent practitioners. Also, the role of the primary care physician (PCP) or some other "gatekeeper" (perhaps an advanced nurse practitioner [ANP]) crystallized as the underpinning for the anticipated success of cost containment, cost reduction, and improvement in coordination of care. The PCPs and ANPs became the fulcrum of managed care (really the *financial management of health care*) and grew to be the single greatest force in the attempt to reduce health care costs. In the year 2000, it is estimated that 50 percent of the population will be registered in some form of managed care plan (Montefiore Medical Center, 1994).

As a result of the independent actions taken by the industry, health care costs rose only by a single digit. Albeit, the inflation rate for the cost of living was still significantly below health care costs, it was the first time in many years that the cost of health care was not rising in the double-digit range.

Reported in *Modern Healthcare*, October, 1994, was the rather startling fact that the hospital producer price index (PPI) for September, 1993, through September, 1994, was 3.4 percent. Physician PPI was reported to have increased 0.1 percent in August, 1994, but dropped a like amount in September, 1994. It appears the inflationary rate that was a significant issue in health care reform may in fact have corrected itself. Given that the cost of health care appears to be under control, one could expect that the issue of *universal* coverage will be the focal point of reform activities.

### Why Is Universal Coverage Still an Issue?

If one believes all the reports of the improvement in diminishing health care costs, then why is universal coverage still a rallying cry? Because a significant number of Americans are without health care insurance and subsequently forego needed health care services. Published in *Modern Healthcare* (1995) was an article describing a voluntary program instituted at a Virginia hospital where patients who are *un*insured or *under*insured can *work* off their hospital bills. This approach is unique in this era of health care delivery, but very traditional in the United States. It is called bartering and is an effective method to *trade* one service for another. As described in the article, both patients and hospital are winners. Innovative and creative nongovernmental methods to finance health care will continue to proliferate during the later part of the 1990s. It would probably be best if the industry could discover the answer to the problem rather than having the government intervene.

## Medicare and Health Maintenance Organizations

As the post-World War II baby boomers age and become recipients of M/C benefits, the aging process becomes decelerated, and longevity continues to have an upward grade, the federal government searches for ways to reduce M/C expenditures. Based on historical utilization of M/C covered service, the government has legitimate reason for concern. According to the Remington Review (1994, April/May), published in *The Remington Report*, consumption of all M/C covered services has grown from 366 persons served per 1,000 in 1967 to 792 persons served per 1,000 in 1990; this translates to an average payment per beneficiary of $593 in 1967 to $3,743 in 1990. During the same time period, the expenditures for home care rose from 1 to 3.7 percent.

As the government investigates methodologies to limit entitlement, or at least shift part of the cost to the beneficiaries, more informed consumers, who have been paying into the system for most or all of their working lives, are becoming eligible for M/C. They do not want to be, as they perceive, "shortchanged."

With impressive speed and marketing techniques, health maintenance organizations (HMOs) are racing to enroll the heretofore untapped M/C population in their programs. The federal government sees HMOs as a viable solution to the ever-increasing expenditures for M/C covered services. The M/C recipients see the copayment savings (usually 20 percent) as "found money." It would appear there is a win/win/win on the horizon—M/C, taxpayers, and recipients. The big loser will be the independent groups, organizations, alliances, and networks that are not part of, or an actual, HMO.

Are HMOs the answer to reducing M/C expenditures? The jury is still out on the decision, since only about 10 percent of the M/C population is enrolled in an HMO. As one would expect, the western section of the United States (California, Arizona, Nevada, and Hawaii) has the highest M/C HMO enrollment with just over 900,000 enrollees. Also, a recent study by Mathematica Policy Research, funded by the federal government, concluded the government was not attaining the expected monetary savings through M/C HMO enrollment; in fact, the HMO population cost 5.7 percent more in comparison to traditional fee for service (Remington, 1994).

### Home Care Capitation

The thought of capitation is frightening to many home care administrators and financial managers, but it has the very real potential to become the method of payment by *all* payers in the near future. For the most part, the industry has not learned that primary contract methods and variants for capitation have already emerged!

Global capitation is the most common methodology. Under this type of arrangement, an agency is paid a set amount of money per patient per month (PPPM) regardless of the number of beneficiaries consuming service. *Disease specific* capitation is founded on the global premise but encompasses only one disease and spreads the *risk* over the entire enrolled population with the disease. Another variant is *active patient* capitation, where the costs for patients with a specific disease are distributed among those *actively* using services. This last capitation design could be financially enticing for home care organizations that have costs under control and have resources (finances and personnel) to specialize in specific treatment modalities (. . . home health line, 1995).

## Mergers, Acquisitions, and Consolidation of Health Care Organizations

As organizations jockeyed for position in the race to maintain viability in the coming era of health care reform, there was an ideologic transformation of the industry. The notion of cost efficiency and cost effectiveness had long been in vogue for the health care industry, but words and phrases like economy of scale, deep discounting, reengineering the work force, and reduction in force (RIF), which had been considered heresy, now glide smoothly off the tongues of administrators. The era of transformation was, and is, upon the industry.

As any industry goes through transformation and renaissance, there are concerns about monopolies forming, restraint of trade, deterioration of quality, and unethical business practices. Are these legitimate concerns for health care as it continues its renaissance? Absolutely.

Reported in the *Wall Street Journal* (1994) were the activities of Columbia/HCA Healthcare Corporation. In part, the article describes how Columbia/HCA has "bought, bargained and battered its way past obstacles to lash together a *powerful* (emphasis added) 16 facility network. . . ." Columbia/HCA currently owns one in four hospitals in Florida and is continually broadening its range of services to encompass all *facets* of health care delivery. Since the 1994 *Wall Street Journal* article, Columbia/HCA has acquired *HealthTrust, AMI,* and *NME.* The company boasts that 95 percent of the population is within twenty minutes of one of its facilities.

Heretofore, the Federal Trade Commission (FTC) has focused its examination on hospital mergers and how the mergers affect in-patient care. Therefore the interest of the FTC has not been piqued by any one company, such as Columbia/HCA, diversifying into the spectrum of health care services that include home care. ". . . And after the owner of a local home-health care company was killed, Columbia swooped in to purchase the business from her estate . . ." (Tomsho, 1994). That does not mean the FTC is unaware of Columbia/HCA. In 1993, it did block the acquisition of one hospital, citing the company would control two of the three hospitals in a local area.

## Price Cutting

Tactics used by predatory organizations are questionable at a minimum. The expected gains and results from these practices are transparent—increased market share and elimination of the competition.

Price cutting is but one tactic. In the retail business world it is called a loss leader; put an item on the shelf at or below cost to get the consumer (in this case payer) in the door, then cultivate more profitable sales. In the health care arena the approach is to undercut the competitors' prices for diagnostic and treatment procedures, in-patient stays, same-day surgeries, or home care. Once a significant portion of the market is under the control of one provider, then the provider drives reimbursement rates. The national conglomerates do have the distinct advantage of economy of scale and subscribe to a cavalier attitude when courting new payers. This will be incremental business, so what is there to lose? Undercutting prices effectively chokes the revenue stream of the competitors until the circumstances are intolerable and two options are available—acquisition or termination of the business.

Do home care organizations need to worry? Absolutely!

## HOME CARE IN THE "NEW ORDER"

If the days of receiving health care in an acute care hospital are coming to an end, alternative avenues of care must be made available. Thus the importance, impact, and value of home care in the new order of health care is becoming more and more apparent. If patient's rights and wishes have any influence on point-of-care decisions, then home care is not only an alternative but the preference of many individuals.

## Gearing Up for the Future

The increase in the number of certified home health agencies (CHHAs) in the United States has been striking—1,014 in an eighteen-month period between June, 1992, and December, 1993. The largest number of new agencies was found in Louisiana, which made that state third in the nation for number of CHHAs. Oklahoma saw a 66 percent increase during the same time period. Neither state has certificate of need (CON) or licensure requirements (The Remington Review, 1994, April/May). Although the east and west coast did not add the number of agencies that other areas of the nation did, two states, New York and California, were the dominant forces in home care spending. Between the two they accounted for 56 percent of *all* home care expenditures (The Remington Review, 1994, April/May). Do these numbers and percentages appear to be the result of questionable business practices in the industry? Suspect business principles could have influenced this growth. But the stronger likelihood is because the number of hospital days per episode of illness continues to shrink and patients are discharged "sicker and quicker," care must continue outside the hospital—in the home, *subacute care facility* (SACF), or some other venue where support and physical attention can be provided. Subacute care facility is the term in use today to describe what at one time was called a convalescent home. The SACF is designed to provide a minimal amount of skilled care for a patient whose acuity no longer justifies hospitalization. Usually this is a self-pay arrangement. The adage *the more things change, the more they stay the same* is so true.

## The Business within the Industry

Home care has a long and inspiring history of making an impressive difference in the lives of patients and their families. However, home care has many problems as a business within an industry. For instance, it

- is fragmented
- is decentralized
- has an "arm's length" relationship with the medical community
- has a patient population that is either very old or young and hopelessly ill
- does not have a concrete identity
- is not integrated within any system
- is touch, not technology (Reece, 1994)

Conversely, all that can be seen as negative has a very positive side, which includes

- flexibility
- innovation
- closeness to the public
- ability to lower costs
- perhaps most important, ability to be *primary care based* (Reece, 1994).

As a whole, the home care segment of the industry needs to go beyond the traditional market targets, beyond the boundaries of the "box" of home care, and become the proactive force in shaping how health care reform will affect the patient. Stop to think—if the number of hospital beds is decreasing and the number of persons requiring health care is increasing, there is an extraordinary opportunity for business development. Broadening the services provided to encompass occupational health service, mobile urgent care services, "labs on wheels," and other services and programs that heretofore were only provided within the four walls of a hospital are fertile fields of opportunity. Developing the entrepreneurial talents of the home care industry is not that difficult since it is flexible and able to adjust, realign, and accommodate to change; because that is the milieu it is accustomed to operating in.

The later half of the 1990s and the new millennium will bring incredible opportunities for those within the home care industry and the entire health care sector who have insight, welcome and embrace change, and look to the future with anticipation and energy. For those who do not—get out of the way!

# ABUNDANCE OF STAFF

As traditional health care employment areas such as hospitals continue to downsize their work force and reengineer how care is delivered, there will be an increasing number of professionals who look to nontraditional settings for employment. For professional staff, as described in earlier chapters, home care holds the opportunity to practice in an autonomous, self-directed, rewarding, and fulfilling environment that is guaranteed to hold new experiences and challenges every day.

The United States Department of Commerce reported that employment in the home heath care sector grew 17.6 percent annually between 1990 and 1993. During the same period, employment grew by only 3.8 percent annually for the entire industry (The Remington Review, 1994, April/May). As hospitals reduce in-patient operations, numerous and varied professional, paraprofessional, and nonprofessional staff will be available in the employment marketplace. Even though hospitals will absorb some of the displaced staff into expanded outpatient and ambulatory services, the likelihood that these enhanced services will operate twenty-four hours a day, seven days a week is remote; thus a considerable number of staff will still be available for other service-delivery modalities.

## Staffing Needs for Enhanced Service Delivery Lines

As HHAs broaden their service delivery lines to include home infusion, high-risk maternal child, advanced cardiac care, geriatrics, psychiatry, and so forth, they will require expertise in these areas of clinical practice. Again, the hospital will be an area for technically skilled resources as the transition from inpatient to outpatient occurs.

The role of ANPs remains to be seen in the new era of health care reform. However, with a rather high degree of certainty, there will be a new and extended role for professionals with these types of qualifications.

### Assistants and Technicians

The utilization of assistants and technicians will grow as the need for the licensed professional will be to assess, evaluate, and oversee the care of the patient. The conflict in the number of visits required versus the number of professional resources available can be relieved by increasing the number of ancillary personnel available to the professional staff.

The use of assistants and technicians has the potential to cause a certain degree of discomfort for the professional staff who may feel they are relinquishing "control" of the patient to less skilled care givers. To allay some of the uneasiness, involving the professional staff in the development of job descriptions, performance appraisals, and interviewing processes for candidates will restore some sense of control. Further, if a professional staff member can be routinely teamed with the same assistant, confidence and trust can be built between the two.

From a purely monetary position, the costs associated with the provision of care must be reduced lest home care find itself in the same situation currently faced by hospitals. One means of reducing cost is the utilization of assistants and technicians, *providing* the quality of patient care is not adversely affected and that there is not so much dissatisfaction among the professional staff that the use of assistants and technicians becomes a morale, retention, and recruitment issue.

# AUTOMATION

With one exception, there are many uncertainties for health care providers as health care reform and a new age for health care delivery systems looms on the horizon. That exception is that there will be an exquisite need and demand for automation. Historically the home care sector has carried the heaviest burden in relation to paper requirements. If for no other reason than paper reduction, fully integrated, comprehensive automation is needed in this segment of the industry.

## Automation and Contract Negotiation

Aside from paper reduction, at no other time has one management tool been so critical and integral to the success and survival of an organization. Without reliable and timely management information, agencies will not be able to expediently address cost and service issues. More important, they will be unable to take offensive or defensive actions to alter operations when faced with unexpected opportunities, or worse, reimbursement hardships.

In order to negotiate financially and operationally sound contracts with the wide variety of managed care organizations and HMOs, sophisticated information is required. Michael R. Cohen (1994) wrote, "Clinical information will be used defensively. In today's environment, it is not unusual for a managed care company to have more detailed information about a provider's patient population and service mix than the provider. This gives them the distinct advantage when contracts are being negotiated."

### Automated Patient Outcome Data

Managed care organizations and HMOs will demand patient outcome data before entering into agreements. It was only in late 1994 that the importance of detailed, objective, and measurable patient outcomes came screaming to the forefront of the industry. For many years, patient outcomes were determined by the attainment of goals at the time of discharge. Albeit a start, it was and is far too elementary for the advanced approach of the managed care organizations. To remain competitive in the home care marketplace, agencies will be required to quantify the results of the care rendered (goals) *and* how many *weeks* and *visits* it took to attain those goals. For large complex agencies, automation is the only foreseeable answer. For smaller agencies, the need may not be as pressing, but if accurate and reliable data are the key to survival, then automation unlocks the door for all agencies.

## Electronic Medical Records

The electronic medical record (EMR) is fast becoming the perceived panacea in the quest to reduce costs, improve efficiency, and become part of a paperless business. The needs of the industry are moving faster than the technology available. It is very difficult to comprehend that technology is moving slower than the need! Heretofore, an industry would wait for technology to settle down before embarking on full-scale automation. Today the home care industry is pleading with the computer industry, software and hardware, to develop a truly comprehensive, fully integrated clinical, business, and personnel system that is

- user friendly
- capable of having many user defined functions
- needing little downtime
- able to be modified easily to meet federal and payer requirements
- not antiquated the day after it is installed
- of course, be priced within reason

It's an interesting challenge for both sides.

The days of shared data bases and service bureaus for home care automation are rapidly coming to an end. Agencies require information almost as it is becoming available and service bureaus are not designed to provide *timely* information. No matter the size of an agency, or at what stage of automation the agency is in, management is well-advised to have dedicated, on-site information system (IS) personnel. The role of IS is evolving and growing as needs continue to escalate for information and assistance with the interpretation of that information.

## Unrealistic Expectations

If the home care industry waits for the *perfect* product, as is so often the case among health care providers and professionals, the industry will truly have "missed the boat."

As important as price is in this era of cost containment, it is truly *penny wise and pound foolish* to put off implementation of a system waiting for perfection. Appreciable time will pass before there is one system that answers all the unique needs of home care. Until that time, it is better to purchase and interface stand-alone systems that do a superlative job at one or more of the needs while the computer industry continues to do the research and development of the *perfect* system.

## CONCLUSION

Traditionally Americans do not demonstrate moderation, but we are well-known for our extremism—witness the chaotic activity in the industry. Attempting to remake, retool, and redesign an entire industry with literally one stroke of the pen is yet another example of our zealous, and unfortunately impatient, nature. The American public is not likely to respond well, if at all, to the notion they will be *told* who, where, and how they will receive health care. Given the fact that health care spending is well on its way to being self-controlled, one might expect that the passionate rhetoric of *health care for all* will soon become a whisper in the halls of Congress. What the 104th Congress will do about the changing tide toward health care remains to be seen, but the business of health care will certainly change. There are many questions still to be answered.

- How and where will health care be delivered?
- Who will manage the care that is delivered?
- What operational restructuring will be needed for organizations to survive?

They are not easy questions to answer and the wrong answers can truly be lethal.

## REFERENCES

Cohen, M. R. (1994). Positioning for communitywide care. *Prospectus.* San Bernadino, CA: Health Data Sciences Corp.

*Health Systems Review.* New GOP health chairman looks to private sector for answers. January/February 1995. pp. 8–11.

. . . *home health line.* (January 9,1995). With "active patient" capitation you could score profits on even the most expensive patients. pp. 3–4.

*Modern Healthcare.* (October 17, 1994). For the record. p.16.

*Modern Healthcare.* (January 23, 1995). Hospital lets patients work to pay bills they can't afford. pp. 18–19.

Montefiore Medical Center. (1994). *Positioning Montefiore for Managed Care.* Bronx, NY: Montefiore Medical Center.

Reece, R. (1994). Community-based health measurement program: a new opportunity for the home health industry. *Remington Report,* April/May. pp. 19–23.

Remington, L. (1994). Medicare HMO enrollment rising. *Remington Report,* April/May. pp. 32–33.

The Remington Review. (1994). Home care growth outpacing industry. *Remington Report,* April/May. p. 13.

The Remington Review. (1994). Home care industry. *Remington Report*, April/May. pp. 1–5.

The Remington Review. (1994). Medicare program expenditures. *Remington Report*, April/May. p. 13.

Solovy, A. (1995). Predicting the unpredictable. *Hospitals and Health Networks*, January 5, 1995, pp. 26–29.

Tomsho, R. (July 12, 1994). Medical tiger giant hospital chain uses tough tactics to push fast growth. *The Wall Street Journal*, pp. A1, A6.

## Suggested Reading

Braunstein, M. L. (1994). Electronic patient records: a key to the managed care challenge? *Remington Report*, August/September, pp. 14–16.

Coriaty, B. (1994). The next generation in computer technology has arrived. *The Remington Report*. June/July, pp. 24–29.

The Week In Health Care. (October 19, 1994). Tomorrow the world. *Modern Healthcare*. pp. 2,3,10,14.

# LIST OF ABBREVIATIONS

| | | | |
|---|---|---|---|
| A&G | administration and general | ECS | electronic claims submission |
| A/P | accounts payable | EMR | electronic medical record |
| A/R | accounts receivable | FFS | fee for service |
| ADC | average daily census | FI | fiscal intermediary |
| ADN | assistant director of nursing | FT | full-time |
| ADT | admission, discharge, transfer | FTC | Federal Trade Commission |
| ALP | assisted living program | FTE | full-time equivalent |
| ANP | advanced nurse practitioner | FY | fiscal year |
| ANS | administrative nursing supervisor | GAAP | generally accepted accounting principles |
| BSW | bachelor's in social work | GL | general ledger |
| CCO | chief clinical officer | HCFA | Health Care Financing Administration |
| CEO | chief executive officer | | |
| CFO | chief financial officer | HHA | home health aids |
| CHAP | Community Healthcare Accreditation Program | HHA | home health care agency |
| | | HHC | Health and Hospital Corporation |
| CHHA | certified home health agency | | |
| CNA | certified nursing assistant | HME | home medical equipment |
| CON | certificate of need | HMO | health maintenance organization |
| COPs | conditions of participation | | |
| CORF | Comprehensive Outpatient Rehabilitation Facility | IRS | Internal Revenue Service |
| | | IS | information systems |
| COTA | certified occupational therapy assistant | IV | intravenous |
| | | JCAHO | Joint Commission for Accreditation of Healthcare Organizations |
| CPA | certified public accountant | | |
| CPR | cardiopulmonary resuscitation | | |
| | | LBS | Ladies Benevolent Society |
| CQI | continuous quality improvement | LCC | lower of cost or charges |
| | | LOS | length of stay |
| CSW | certification of social work | LPN | licensed practical nurse |
| DCN | direct care nurse | LTHHCP | Long Term Home Health Care Programs |
| DME | durable medical equipment | | |
| DoH | Department of Health | LVN | licensed vocational nurse |
| DPS | director of patient services | M/A | Medicaid |
| DRG | diagnosis related grouping | M/C | Medicare |
| DSS | Department of Social Service | MBA | master's in business administration |
| EAP | employee assistance program | | |

| | | | |
|---|---|---|---|
| MCH | maternal child health | PIP | periodic interim payment |
| MCO | managed care organization | POC | plan of care |
| MetLife | Metropolitan Life Insurance Company | PPI | producer price index |
| | | PPO | preferred provider organization |
| MIS | management information system | | |
| | | PPPM | per patient per month |
| MSW | master's in social work | PPS | prospective payment system |
| MSW | medical social work | PS&R | Provider Statistical and Reimbursement System |
| MUT | maximum utilization threshold | | |
| | | PSM | patient service manager |
| NAHC | National Association for Home Care | PT | part-time |
| | | PT | physical therapy |
| NPR | Notice of Provider Reimbursement | PTA | physical therapy assistant |
| | | QI | quality improvement |
| OBRA-80 | Omnibus Budget Reconciliation Act of 1980 | QM | quality management |
| | | RFI | request for information |
| OBRA-81 | Omnibus Budget Reconciliation Act of 1981 | RHHI | Regional Home Health Intermediary |
| OBRA-87 | Omnibus Reconciliation Act of 1987 | RIF | reduction in force |
| | | RM | risk management |
| OBRA-90 | Omnibus Reconciliation Act of 1990 | RN | registered nurse |
| | | RT | respiratory therapy |
| OBRA-93 | Omnibus Reconciliation Act of 1993 | S/O | significant other |
| | | SACF | subacute care facility |
| OHS | occupational health services | SN | skilled nursing |
| OSHA | Occupational Safety and Health Administration | SNF | skilled nursing facility |
| | | SP | speech pathology |
| OT | occupational therapy | T.O. | table of organization |
| OT | overtime | TQM | total quality management |
| P/L | profit/loss | UB | universal bill |
| PC | personal computer | UPS | uninterruptible power supply |
| PCP | primary care physician | UR | utilization review |
| PCW | patient care worker | VNA | Visiting Nurse Association |
| PHO | physician-hospital organization | VNSNY | Visiting Nurse Service of New York |

# INDEX

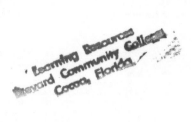